Heat stress and what it means for people's health

By C.Miya

ABSTRACT

Global warming has led to renewed interest in the occurrence of heat stress in the population along with its determinants and consequences. Heat stress can create unsafe working conditions and affect the health of workers. Heat waves are also unsafe and in 2003 led to many avoidable deaths in Europe. Most heat stress research has been conducted in high-income countries in temperate latitudes. This leaves knowledge gaps regarding heat stress and its effects for tropical settings.

Thailand is a tropical developing country where average temperatures have increased over the last 50 years and further increase is expected. Heat stress has been shown to be a serious problem in a variety of Thai workplaces. But several important public health questions remain and they are the focus of this thesis. The questions are as follows: are there any health impacts of heat stress i) on Thai workers? ii) on the overall population in Thailand? iii) expected for the Thai population in future due to the projected increase of temperature?

To answer these research questions, five studies were carried out. They investigate the occurrence of heat stress and its association with various health outcomes, including death. The first four studies use heat exposure and morbidity data from a large national Thai Cohort Study (TCS) covering the period 2005 to 2009. The fifth study uses national weather and mortality data covering 1999 to 2008.

The first study explores the relationship between self-reported heat stress and psychological distress and overall health status of Thai workers using TCS data. There was a strong association between heat stress and worse mental health outcomes among workers.

The second study uses TCS data on heat stress and occupational injury among Thai workers. The evidence connects heat stress and occupational injury and also identifies several factors that increase heat exposure (male sex, rural residence, physical job).

The third study relates heat stress and incident kidney disease amongst Thai workers using longitudinal TCS data that documented prolonged heat exposure. Heat stress was a significant risk factor for kidney disease among male workers, especially physical workers age 35 years or more.

The fourth study shows that health and wellbeing decreased (low energy, emotional problems, and low life satisfaction) as more heat stress interfered with daily activities (sleeping, daily travel, work, housework and exercise). So heat stress has an adverse health impact on the overall population.

The final study shows that Thai mortality from 1999 to 2008, adjusted for weather and air pollution, varied by air temperature. A U-shaped association between monthly maximum temperature and mortality was found for each season (hot, wet, and cold), and each region (North, Northeast, South, and Centre). The 4 degrees Celsius increase in temperature from climate change, as expected by 2100, could increase annual heat-related deaths by 32,000 as well as increasing other impacts on health and well-being.

The health impact information in this thesis points to the need to improve health surveillance and public awareness regarding risks of heat stress in Thailand.

TABLE OF CONTENTS

PUBLICATIONS AND PRESENTATIONS

This thesis contains five published articles in peer-reviewed journal and five presentations at international conferences.

Peer reviewed journal articles:

1. Tawatsupa B, Lim LL-Y, Kjellstrom T, Seubsman S, Sleigh A, the Thai Cohort Study team (2010) The association between overall health, psychological distress, and occupational heat stress among a large national cohort of 40,913 Thai workers. *Global Health Action* 3. DOI: 10.3402/gha.v3i0.5034.

2. Tawatsupa B, Yiengprugsawan V, Kjellstrom T, Berecki-Gisolf J, Seubsman S, Sleigh A (2013) The association between heat stress and occupational injury among Thai workers: finding of the Thai Cohort Study. *Industrial Health* 51.

3. Tawatsupa B, Lim LL-Y, Kjellstrom T, Seubsman S, Sleigh A, the Thai Cohort Study Team (2012). Association between occupational heat stress and kidney disease among 37,816 workers in the Thai Cohort Study (TCS). *Journal of Epidemiology* 22. DOI: 10.2188/jea.JE20110082.

4. Tawatsupa B, Yiengprugsawan V, Kjellstrom T, Seubsman S, Sleigh A, the Thai Cohort Study Team (2012) Heat stress, health, and wellbeing: findings from a large national cohort of Thai adults. *BMJ Open* 2. DOI: 10.1136/bmjopen-2012-001396.

5. Tawatsupa B, Dear K, Kjellstrom T, Sleigh A (2012) The association between temperature and mortality in tropical middle income Thailand from 1999 to 2008. *International Journal of Biometeorology.* DOI: 10.1007/s00484-012-0597-8.

Conference Presentations

1. Benjawan Tawatsupa (2010) "The association between overall health, psychological distress and occupational heat stress among a large national cohort of 40,913 Thai workers". The International Conference Workshop on "Livelihood and Health Impacts of the Climate Change: Community Adaptation Strategies", Khon Khen University, Khon Khen, Thailand. 24-25 August 2010 (Oral presentation).

2. Benjawan Tawatsupa (2010) "The association between overall health, psychological distress and occupational heat stress among a large national cohort of 40,913 Thai workers". Conference on Health and Mortality Transitions in East and Southeast Asia, Australian Demographic and Social Research Institute (ADSRI), The Australian National University, Canberra, 25-27 October 2010 (Oral presentation).

3. Benjawan Tawatsupa (2011) "The association between weather variations and air pollution conditions and mortality in tropical and developing countries - Thailand from 1999 to 2008". Greenhouse 2011 Conference, Cairns, Australia. 4-8 April 2011 (Poster presentation).

4. Benjawan Tawatsupa (2011) The association between workplace heat stress and kidney disease among more than 30,000 men and women in the Thai Cohort Study (TCS)". The International Congress of Biometeorology (ICB2011), Auckland University, Auckland, New Zealand. 5-9 December 2011 (Oral presentation).

5. Benjawan Tawatsupa (2012) "The association between weather variations and mortality in Thailand". CCI Climate Change PhD EXPO 2012, Australian National University, Canberra, Australia. 16 March 2012 (Poster presentation)

I was the corresponding author who took primary responsibility for overall management of drafting process, data analysis and responded to comments from journal editors and reviewers for all five published papers. The structure of published articles is preserved in each chapter. As each paper included contributions from all co-authors, the statements of candidate's contribution are given in Table 1.

Table 1 Candidate's contribution for each paper presented in this thesis

Chapter*	Publication title	Journal	Year of publication	No. of authors	Candidate contribution		
					Conception & design	Analysis & interpretation	Drafting & revising
Chapter 3 Heat stress and mental health	The association between overall health, psychological distress, and occupational heat stress among a large national cohort of 40,913 Thai workers	Global Health Action	Published 2010	5	√	√	√
Chapter 4 Heat stress and occupational injury	The association between heat stress and occupational injury among Thai workers: finding of the TCS	Industrial Health	Published 2013	5	√	√	√
Chapter 5 Heat stress and kidney disease	Association between occupational heat stress and kidney disease among 37,816 workers in the Thai Cohort Study (TCS)	Journal of Epidemiology	Published 2012	5	√	√	√
Chapter 6 Heat stress and well-being	Heat stress, health, and wellbeing: findings from a large national cohort of Thai adults	BMJ Open	Published 2012	6	√	√	√
Chapter 7 Heat stress and mortality	The association between temperature and mortality in tropical middle income Thailand from 1999 to 2008	International Journal of Biometeoro-logy	Published 2012	4	√	√	√

*The structure of published articles is preserved in each chapter

CONTRIBUTION DECLARATIONS FOR

PUBLICATION

Paper 1: Tawatsupa B, Lim LL-Y, Kjellstrom T, Seubsman S, Sleigh A, the Thai Cohort Study team (2010) The association between overall health, psychological distress, and occupational heat stress among a large national cohort of 40,913 Thai workers. *Global Health Action* 3. DOI: 10.3402/gha.v3i0.5034.

Candidate and co-authors' contribution: I prepared a draft paper, literature review and performed the data analysis under supervision of LL. LL advised on data analysis and data interpretations. TK had the initial idea for the heat stress study. SS and AS conceived and executed the Thai Cohort Study. LL, TK, SS, and AS supported valuable comments and evaluated the final version of manuscript. AS supervised development of work and supported for revising and editing paper for the final version. All authors contributed to and approved the final version to be published.

Authors' approval: each author certifies that this level of contribution by the candidate indicated above is appropriate and that permission is granted for this paper to be included in the candidate's thesis.

Authors' name	Signature	Date
Corresponding author (Candidate): Benjawan Tawatsupa	*Benjawan Tawatsupa*	2 –10 –2012
Author 2: Lynette L-Y Lim		2/10/n.
Author 3: Tord Kjellstrom		4.10.12
Author 4: Sam-ang Seubsman	*Sam-ang Seubsman*	8.10.12
Author 5: Adrian Sleigh		2 –10 – 2012

4

Paper 2: Tawatsupa B, Yiengprugsawan V, Kjellstrom T, Berecki-Gisolf J, Seubsman S, Sleigh A (2013) The association between heat stress and occupational injury among Thai workers: finding of the Thai Cohort Study. Industrial Health 51.

Candidate and co-authors' contribution: I had a substantial contribution to the conception and study design of this paper. I drafted the manuscript. I did the literature search, and statistical analysis. AS assisted with the writing and interpretation. SS and AS conceived and executed the Thai Cohort Study. VY, J B-G, TK, SS, and AS gave comments and feedback for the final version. All authors contributed to and approved the final version.

Authors' approval: each author certifies that this level of contribution by the candidate indicated above is appropriate and that permission is granted for this paper to be included in the candidate's thesis.

Authors' name	Signature	Date
Corresponding author (Candidate): Benjawan Tawatsupa	*Benjawan Tawatsupa*	2-10-2012
Author 2: Vasoontara Yiengprugsawan		2/10/2012
Author 3: Tord Kjellstrom		3/10/12
Author 4: Janneke Berecki-Gisolf		4/10/2012
Author 5: Sam-ang Seubsman		8/10/12
Author 6: Adrian Sleigh		2-10·2012

5

Paper 3: Tawatsupa B, Lim LL-Y, Kjellstrom T, Seubsman S, Sleigh A, the Thai Cohort Study Team (2012). Association between occupational heat stress and kidney disease among 37,816 workers in the Thai Cohort Study (TCS). Journal of Epidemiology 22. DOI: 10.2188/jea.JE20110082.

Candidate and co-authors' contribution: I conducted a literature review from the international studies and those in Thailand. I wrote a draft paper and did the statistical analysis under supervision of LL. LL had initial idea for kidney disease study and helped in data interpretation. SS and AS conceived and executed the Thai Cohort Study. LL, TK, SS, and AS supported comments and suggestions for the final version of manuscript. I revised the manuscript under supervision of AS who supported for the revision and editing paper. All authors contributed to the manuscript at all stages and approved the final version.

Authors' approval: each author certifies that this level of contribution by the candidate indicated above is appropriate and that permission is granted for this paper to be included in the candidate's thesis.

Authors' name	Signature	Date
Corresponding author (Candidate): Benjawan Tawatsupa	*Benjawan Tawatsupa*	2 - 10-2012
Author 2: Lynette L-Y Lim		2/10/12
Author 3: Tord Kjellstrom		3/10/12
Author 4: Sam-ang Seubsman		8/10/12
Author 5: Adrian Sleigh		2-10-2012

Paper 4: Tawatsupa B, Yiengprugsawan V, Kjellstrom T, Seubsman S, Sleigh A, the Thai Cohort Study Team (2012) Heat stress, health, and wellbeing: findings from a large national cohort of Thai adults. *BMJ Open* 2. DOI: 10.1136/bmjopen-2012-001396.

Candidate and co-authors' contribution: I and VY conceptualised the analysis for this paper with contributions from all authors. I wrote the first draft manuscript and did the literature search. I also did statistical analysis under supervision of VY. VY supervised development of work and help in data interpretation. SS and AS conceived and executed the Thai Cohort Study. TK, VY, SS and AS assisted in writing and interpretation. All authors contributed to and approved the final version.

Authors' approval: each author certifies that this level of contribution by the candidate indicated above is appropriate and that permission is granted for this paper to be included in the candidate's thesis.

Authors' name	Signature	Date
Corresponding author (Candidate): Benjawan Tawatsupa	*Benjawan Tawatsupa*	2-10-2012
Author 2: Vasoontara Yiengprugsawan	*V. Yiengprug*	3/10/2012
Author 3: Tord Kjellstrom	*Tord Kjell*	3/10/12
Author 4: Sam-ang Seubsman	*Sam-ang Subman*	8/10/12
Author 5: Adrian Sleigh	*A C Sgh*	2-10-2012

Paper 5: Tawatsupa B, Dear K, Kjellstrom T, Sleigh A (2012) The association between temperature and mortality in tropical middle income Thailand from 1999 to 2008. *International Journal of Biometeorology.* (Special Issue: ICB 2011 - Students / New Professionals). DOI: 10.1007/s00484-012-0597-8.

Candidate and co-authors' contribution: I did the literature search and wrote the draft manuscript. I did the fieldwork and executed all data using in this study from four National databases of Thailand. I also analysed data using advanced analyses under technical and material support from KD and TK. KD and AS supervised the statistical analysis and described the analytical model. AS edited the manuscript and assisted with data interpretation. KD, AS and TK supported valuable comments and suggestions for the final version. I revised the manuscript under supervision of AS and KD who supported for the revision and editing paper. All authors contributed to the conception and design and approved the final version.

Authors' approval: each author certifies that this level of contribution by the candidate indicated above is appropriate and that permission is granted for this paper to be included in the candidate's thesis.

Authors' name	Signature	Date
Corresponding author (Candidate): Benjawan Tawatsupa	*Benjawan Tawatsupa*	2 – 10 –2012
Author 2: Keith Dear	*(signature)*	3- 10- 12
Author 3: Tord Kjellstrom	*(signature)*	4. 10. 19
Author 4: Adrian Sleigh	*(signature)*	2- 10 -2012

CHAPTER 1: INTRODUCTION

This chapter presents an overview of the heat stress problem and public health concern about impacts of heat stress on human health. Then unanswered questions from existing studies and the rationale for this study are discussed. The research questions and conceptual framework including aims and objectives have been set up to seek a more comprehensive understanding of heat stress and human health impacts in Thailand. The last section of this chapter describes the thesis structure.

1.1 Background

Over the last two decades interest has grown in the impact of climate change on human health and well-being. It was reported by the Intergovernmental Panel on Climate Change (IPCC) in 2007 that the global average temperature increased by about 0.74°C during the last century (1906-2005) and is likely to continue to increase in the future (IPCC 2007). The ongoing increase in global average temperature, combined with an increase in weather variability, is likely to increase the intensity, frequency and duration of extreme weather and climate events such as heat waves, droughts and floods (McMichael et al. 2003). Also, the rising average temperature will lead to an increase in the number of hot days and warm nights (IPCC 2007).

Heat stress has become an important issue in public health and epidemiology, especially since the severe European heat waves in 2003 (Kovats and Hajat 2008). Since then many researchers have studied the relationship between heat stress and mortality in various countries (Confalonieri et al. 2007; McMichael et al. 2008; Gosling et al. 2009a). Several studies revealed that an increasing temperature is likely to increase incidences of heat-related illness, and deaths (McGeehin and Mirabelli 2001; Kovats and Hajat 2008; Basu 2009; Baccini et al. 2011; Ye et al. 2012).

Recently, studies of heat stress have drawn attention to adverse health effects among workers. The international multi-centre health research and prevention program "High Occupational Temperature Health and Productivity Suppression (HOTHAPS)" has developed many research projects focusing on the effects of heat exposure on working people (Kjellstrom et al. 2009a). The projects focus on climate change and its potential to exacerbate occupational heat-related risks such as chronic diseases, mental health problems, occupational injuries, and poor work performance (Kjellstrom et al. 2009a; Kjellstrom and Crowe 2011; Ingole et al. 2012).

The human body is capable of maintaining its core temperature at around 37°C by balancing the body effects of heat gain and heat loss (Parsons 2003). The natural methods for heat loss used by humans include convection, conduction, radiation, and evaporation (Parsons 2003). Only evaporation of sweat will lower body temperature in such an extremely hot environment exceeding body temperature and it will lead to loss of body water and electrolytes. If there is high humidity, evaporation will be reduced and will become a less effective cooling mechanism (Parsons 2003). The combination of high temperature and high humidity together with body physical exertion will lead to sweating, and then dehydration can overwhelm the body's coping mechanisms leading to heat-related illness and even death (MMWR 2008).

Heat stress has acute and chronic effects on human health. The acute effects are heat-related illness including heat rash, heat fatigue, heat cramps, heat exhaustion, heat stroke, or even deaths (Bouchama and Knochel 2002). Among chronic effects, heat stress can increase risks of cardiovascular illnesses, respiratory illnesses, diabetes, and kidney disease (McMichael et al. 2003; Kovats and Hajat 2008; Kjellstrom et al. 2010). Also, heat stress can increase risk of injuries and disruption to well-being (Riedel 2004; Kjellstrom 2009b; Kjellstrom et al. 2010) . Final outcomes may include reduced work productivity and increased risk of psychological distress (Wyndham 1965; Kjellstrom et al. 2010; Kjellstrom and Crowe 2011)

Several epidemiological studies have investigated the association between temperature and mortality. The reports suggest that the projected increase in the global average temperature from climate change, accompanied by an expected increase in weather variability, will lead to an overall increase in the number of deaths due to heat-related deaths and also a decrease in the number of cold-related deaths (Confalonieri et al. 2007). To confirm and consolidate our knowledge on the health effects of climate change there is a need for more studies on the association between heat stress and human health outcomes. These studies should focus on how the existing heat-health relationship may be affected by climate change (Martens 1998; Kovats and Hajat 2008; Gosling et al. 2009a). The studies can also address some important unanswered questions and these are considered below.

1.2 Unanswered questions about heat stress and human health

There are two main knowledge gaps about heat stress effects on human health. First, there is little information about health impacts of heat stress in tropical and developing countries (World Health Organization 2010). Secondly, there is a general lack of evidence about the health impacts of heat stress in working populations (Kjellstrom et al. 2009a; Kjellstrom et al. 2009b).

Several studies on heat stress and its impacts on health have been conducted, but these were mostly in developed and non-tropical countries (Kjellstrom 2009b). This leaves unanswered questions about the effects of warmer weather in tropical and developing countries where very high heat in tropical zones will become even more extreme and more thermally stressful (Kjellstrom 2009b). Also, the air temperature in urban areas of developing countries is expected to increase drastically as a result of the urban heat island effect caused by ongoing industrial development and urbanisation (Oke 1973). If there are no heat prevention or mitigation measures, a rising population in urban areas due to urbanisation of developing countries and aging of the population may lead over time to increased adverse health impacts (McMichael et al. 1998; Campbell-Lendrum and Corvalan 2007).

Also, heat stress can cause a serious occupational injury and ill-health among workers who are exposed to hot and humid work environments (Kjellstrom et al. 2009b). The original report from the heat wave in France in August 2003 documented almost 1,000 additional deaths in the age range 20-60 years (Hémon D and Jougla E 2003).

This age group includes people in the workforce who may be exposed to heavy labour outdoors during hot weather most of the year (Kjellstrom et al. 2009b). With global warming such workers are going to be exposed to very high heat even more frequently, leading to prolonged heat stress without sufficient heat protection and prolonged dehydration (Kjellstrom and Weaver 2009). For these reasons, research on heat stress in the workplace is important, in particular for tropical developing countries.

1.3 Rationale for studying heat stress effects in Thailand

Although several studies on heat and its human impact have shown an association between heat stress and health in many non-tropical developed countries, there are only a few studies conducted in tropical developing countries including Thailand. We lack information that can be used for health impact assessment of climate change in such a setting, which covers a large proportion of the global population. Indeed about 40% of the world's population lives in the tropics, and this proportion is expected to reach 55% by 2050 (McNeil 2009).

Thailand is a middle income tropical country in Southeast Asia with around 65 million people. Following rapid urbanisation, currently around 46% of the Thai population live in urban areas and it is predicted that by 2030 this will be more than 60% (National Statistical Office 2011). Social and economic transitions in Thailand over the last 30 years led to an increase in number of working population in the manufacturing and service sectors (Kelly et al. 2010). More than 39 million people are now in the Thai workforce of which more than 16 million are agricultural workers (National Statistical Office 2012).

As Thailand is located in a tropical zone both air temperature and humidity are high, particularly during the hottest seasons (Meteorological Development Bureau 2012). From 1951 to 2003, the monthly mean maximum temperature in Thailand increased by 0.56°C and the monthly mean minimum temperature increased even more, by 1.44°C (Limsakul and Goes 2008).

In addition, a further increase in air temperature associated with global warming is anticipated in Thailand (Thai Meteorological Department 2007). Warming trends in maximum and minimum temperatures have been found and the number of days with high maximum temperature have significantly increased (Thai Meteorological Department 2007). In the future, temperature increase as a result of climate change may increase adverse health effects among Thai population.

A study of occupational heat stress in Thailand by Langkulsen et al. (2010) indicated that heat stress in Thailand is a very serious problem ("extreme caution" or "danger") in a wide variety of work settings. They tested a pottery factory, a power plant, a knife manufacturing site, a construction site, and an agricultural site. Another study found that salt production workers in Thailand worked under heat stress where average temperature ±SEM (standard error of the mean) in the working environment was 33.8±0.95°C and those workers who worked under heat stress were more likely to have heat symptoms compared to unexposed group (Jakreng 2010).

As noted above, heat stress is already a problem in Thailand and there is a need to be more concerned for occupational heat stress problem among Thai workers. There is already a large number of industrial workers exposed to excessive heat; they fill demanding jobs and ongoing climate change will lead to even higher heat exposures for such workers, especially likely to affect poor people in labouring occupations.

To date, climate change and some of its expected health effects have received limited attention in Thailand. Existing studies include investigation of the health impacts of heat stress in Chiang Mai province in Northern Thailand (Pudpong and Hajat 2011), and study of temperature-associated mortality in Chiang Mai and Bangkok (McMichael et al. 2008). More information is needed on the association of heat stress and potential health outcomes among the general Thai population covering those residing in various parts of the country subject to different sub-climates (inland North and Northeast, tropical Centre, and equatorial South).

1.4 Research questions, aim and conceptual framework

There are three research questions including:

1. Are there any health impacts from heat stress in Thai workers?
2. Are there any health impacts of heat stress on the overall Thai population?
3. Are these health impacts expected to increase due to climate change and the projected increase of temperature?

Therefore, the Aim of this thesis is to investigate the association between heat stress and health outcomes in Thailand, now and in the future.

Health is defined by World Health Organization (WHO) as *"a state of complete physical, mental and social well-being and not merely the absence of disease or infirmity"* (World Health Organization 1946). Reflecting this WHO definition, in this thesis four health outcomes from heat stress are selected to present an holistic account of health impacts from climate change. These include physical health outcomes (heat-related injury and kidney disease), mental health outcomes (heat-related psychological distress), well-being outcomes (heat stress interfering in daily activities and affecting people's feeling of life satisfaction), and overall heat-related deaths.

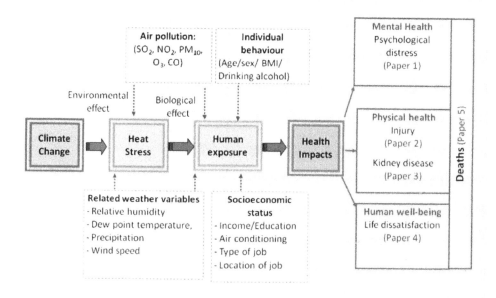

Figure 1.1 Conceptual framework for effects of heat stress on human health in Thailand

The conceptual framework of this thesis for health effects of heat stress is shown in Figure 1.1. The health impact pathway for heat stress involves the linkages of human exposure to heat stress and resulting health outcomes. This thesis also explores the related factors that can modify heat stress effects on human health such as the environment (weather variables and air pollution), individual behaviour, and socioeconomic status of the Thai population.

1.5 Data sources

In this thesis, five studies address the three research question. The first four studies (Chapter 3-6) were conducted using data from a large national health research cohort followed since 2005 (the Thai Cohort Study). The fifth study (Chapter 7) uses four national government datasets on weather, air pollution, mortality, and population covering the period of 1999 to 2008.

1.5.1 The Thai Cohort Study

The Thai Cohort Study (TCS) is a national population based study of Thai adults which is attempting to track and analyse the changing distribution of health patterns and health risks in the Thai population. The cohort was initially recruited from distance learning students enrolled at Sukhothai Thammathirat Open University (STOU) and started with a mail-out questionnaire covering socio-demographic and economic status as well as questions on health behaviours and health outcomes. There were 87,134 students aged 15-87 years who responded from all areas of Thailand in 2005 (Sleigh et al. 2008). Overall, 70% or 60,569 students completed the follow-up study in 2009; they were the same persons as those studied in 2005, and the two data sets have been linked for individual records.

The STOU students in the TCS are represent the overall Thai population reasonably well for geographic location and socioeconomic status for both sexes (Sleigh et al. 2008). The TCS group has a similar sex distribution as the Thai population with a slightly higher proportion of females in the TCS (54.7% vs 50.5%). For age distribution, the TCS group tended to include proportionally more young adults (in range 21-30 year age) than the general population (51.5% vs 23.9%). Among the general Thais, 56.6% had lower than junior higher school education but all TCS members had more school education than that. Close to 19% of Thais reported income less than 3,000 baht per month compared to 11.0% among TCS participants. Geographically, Bangkok and the Central region were most represented among Thais (37.1%) and TCS members (41.4%). The overall similarity of socioeconomic status and geographic representation of the both groups is apparent. However, the differences were the TCS members are younger and better educated than average Thais (Seubsman, et al. 2012). This difference enabled us to gather complex information on heat stress and health outcomes for large numbers by questionnaire.

In the TCS data, the information about heat stress derived from two questions. First, the self-report of heat stress in 2005 using the following question: "During the last twelve months, how often have you experienced high temperatures which make you uncomfortable at work?" Respondents answered on a four point scale – "often", "sometimes", "rarely", and "never". Second, heat stress in 2009 was quantified by five sub-questions as follows: "How often did the hot period this year interfere with your work, sleeping, daily travel, housework, and exercise?" Respondents answered on a five point scale - "everyday", "1-6 times/wk", "1-3 times/month", "never", and "not applicable (N/A) – use air conditioning".

1.5.2 The four national government datasets

The national datasets were obtained from four databases covering weather, air pollution, mortality, and population data from 1999 to 2008 (see Appendix A for additional details of the data). Weather data were obtained from the Thai Meteorological Department for a total of 120 stations in 65 provinces (Meteorological Development Bureau 2010). The data include six weather variables of: mean, minimum, maximum and average dew point temperatures (°C), maximum wind speed (m/s), and average precipitation in 24 hours (mm).

Air pollution data came from the Pollution Control Department for 49 air monitoring stations in 23 provinces (Air Quality and Noise Management Bureau 2010). The monthly maximum and monthly average of daily mean concentrations for five air pollutants are analysed; they included sulphur dioxide (SO_2), nitrogen dioxide (NO_2), carbon monoxide (CO), ozone (O_3), and particulate matter less than 10 micrometre in diameter (PM_{10}).

All-cause mortality data were obtained from individual death records provided by the Bureau of Policy and Strategy, Ministry of Public Health (Bureau of Policy and Strategy 2010a). The Bureau of Policy and Strategy supplied mid-year populations by age-group and sex for each of 76 provinces (Bureau of Policy and Strategy 2010b). These population data enabled calculation of age-sex adjusted death rates (ADR) for each province.

1.6 Objectives

Table 1.1 presents the reasons for selecting the health outcomes and specifies the objectives, data sources and study design. Overall, there are five objectives for five studies to answer the three research questions (see section 1.4 above).

Table 1.1 Reasons for studying the relationship between heat stress
and selected potential health outcomes

Research Questions	Objectives	Reasons	Data source	Study design & Methods
1. Are there any health impacts from heat stress in Thai workers?	1) To identify association between heat stress and mental health in Thai workers	Occupational heat stress is a well-known problem affecting workers health. There are very few recent studies reported the heat stress effects on mental health among workers in tropical developing Thailand.	TCS data: the 1st survey in 2005	Cross-sectional study using logistic regression analysis
	2) To address knowledge gap of heat stress-related occupational injury	Tropical developing countries where heat stress is a problem, excessive expose to heat stress may cause fainting or confusion resulting in a reduction of safety protection and increase occupational injury risks among workers.	TCS data: the 1st survey in 2005	Cross-sectional study using logistic regression analysis
	3) To characterise association between heat stress and incident kidney disease among Thai workers	Kidney disease is a major cause of death among population aged 15 to 65 years (working age group) in Thailand. Kidney disease has been already documented in other studies that it is related to heat stress and prolonged dehydration. It is interesting to explore the association between heat stress at work and kidney disease.	TCS data: baseline survey in 2005 and followed up in 2009	Cross-sectional and prospective cohort study using logistic regression analysis
2. Are there any health impacts of heat stress on the overall Thai population?	4) To examine association between heat stress and holistic health and well-being outcomes	The effects of daily heat stress exposure can have a major influence on human daily activities (sleep, work, daily travel, and household work) but there is limited information regarding the heat stress impact on overall health and wellbeing among Thai population.	TCS data: the 2nd survey in 2009	Cross-sectional study using multinomial logistic regression analysis
	5.1) To investigate relationship between heat stress and mortality	There is a need for study on the relationship between impacts of heat stress on deaths in Thailand. If there is an association between weather and deaths, it is expected that an increase in temperature in the future will contribute to change in pattern of deaths in Thailand and will increase public health problems in the future.	National dataset: weather, air quality, mortality, and population data from 1999 - 2008	Time-series study using Multivariable Fractional Polynomial regression and stepwise multivariable linear regression analysis
3. Are these health impacts expected to increase due to climate change and the projected increase of temperature?	5.2) to estimate heat stress effects on mortality in the future as a result of the expected increase in temperature from climate change.			

For the first research question, "Are there any health impacts from heat stress in Thai workers?" there are three objectives to address the issues.

Objective 1: To identify the association between heat stress and mental health in Thai workers. The data for this study derived from the first survey (in 2005) of a national Thai Cohort Study (TCS). The study population are full-time workers in a cohort as they are commonly exposed to heat by carrying out heavy labour in tropical Thailand.

Objective 2: To address the knowledge gap regarding heat stress-related occupational injury in Thailand. The data of a large national adult cohort, the TCS data in 2005, are analysed to detect epidemiological association between heat stress and occupational injury in the Thai workplace.

Objective 3: To characterise association between heat stress and incident kidney disease among Thai workers. The data are derived from the self-report of a large national cohort (TCS) of Thai workers whose social and physical environment and health outcomes have been followed from 2005 to 2009.

The second research question was "Are there any health impacts of heat stress on the overall Thai population?" Objectives 4 and 5 answer this question.

Objective 4: To examine the association between hot season heat stress (sleeping, work, travel, housework, exercise) and three graded holistic health and well-being outcomes (energy, emotions, life satisfaction) in the Thai population. The data for this study derived from the large national TCS in 2009.

Objective 5: To quantify the association between heat stress and mortality in Thailand by using Thai national datasets from 1999 to 2008. There are two specific study components; the first component investigates the relationship between heat stress and total mortality in Thailand over 10 years (1999 – 2008). The second component projects the heat stress effects on mortality in the future as a result of the expected increase in temperature from climate change. This addresses the last research question; "Are these health impacts expected to increase due to climate change and the projected increase of temperature?"

1.7 Thesis structure

This thesis includes five published papers that collectively address the three research questions and five objectives related to heat stress and health impacts in Thailand. All papers were prepared during my doctoral candidature and are reproduced with the permission of the publishing company and co-authors. The five papers are preserved as published format in Chapter 3-7. There are some chapters providing introduction, literature review, discussion and conclusions that are unpublished.

Chapter 1 Introduction: the thesis begins with a discussion of the background of the heat stress problem and an introduction to the research topic of heat stress and human health impacts. As well, the rationale for studying the health impacts of heat stress is given. This chapter also provides three research questions, an aim, five objectives and a conceptual framework, as well as a study design for identifying the relationships between heat stress and health outcomes. The data sources and objectives are specified and the overall thesis structure is presented.

Chapter 2 Literature review: the review introduces the overall knowledge base on health impacts of heat stress on human health. The physiology and health effects of heat stress are described, especially temperature-related mortality. A critical review summarises previous research findings and knowledge gaps in tropical and developing countries. This chapter tackles the complex problem of heat stress and health impacts on working populations. Then attention turns to Thailand, beginning with the context, awareness and policy for heat stress and human health impacts in Thailand.

Chapter 3 Heat stress and mental health: the working population is vulnerable to heat stress effects if they are often exposed to heat from their job or carry out heavy labour outdoors or indoors without air conditioning. This chapter investigates the association between occupational heat stress and mental health outcomes in Thai workers. This is the first published paper that investigates the association between self-reported heat stress at work and psychological distress and self-rated overall health in working populations. This analysis is a cross-sectional study of the association between self-reported heat stress and mental health by using TCS data in 2005.

Chapter 4 Heat stress and occupational injury: the heat stress impacts may arise from increased mistakes in daily activities and lead to accidental injuries. This second paper reports on the association between heat stress and workplace injury among workers enrolled in the large national TCS in 2005. This study used the TCS data at baseline in 2005 to investigate the relationship between heat stress and occupational injury among Thai workers. This study provides evidence connecting heat stress and occupational injury in tropical Thailand and also identifies several factors that increase heat exposure.

Chapter 5 Heat stress and kidney disease: one interesting health feature of Thai workers in the TCS and the general population is an increase of incident kidney disease. Kidney disease has been reported to be related to heat stress in some studies but not in any reported in tropical and developing countries. Moreover, TCS data are available to investigate the heat stress exposure at baseline in 2005, and also prolonged heat stress exposure in the follow-up study in 2009. Thus, this third paper presents the study of the relationship between self-reported occupational heat stress and incidence of self-reported doctor-diagnosed kidney disease among Thai workers.

Chapter 6 Heat stress and well-being: heat stress not only affects health of workers but also the health of the general population. This fourth paper looks at how heat stress interferes with daily activities (sleeping, daily travel, work, housework and exercise) among the Thai population. It investigates the association between self-reported heat stress and overall health and human well-being. This analysis is a cross-sectional study using multinomial logistic regression analysis of the TCS data in 2009.

Chapter 7 Heat stress and mortality: this last paper is a key study and presents more details of the association between weather variation and mortality in Thailand from 1999 to 2008, taking into account air pollution effects. There are 17 main variables of weather and air pollution, and age-sex adjusted death rates (ADRs) are health outcomes. There are around one million death counts during the 10-year period in the 13 provinces where weather and air pollution data are available. Multivariable fractional polynomial regression is used to create the best transformations for weather variables and air pollutants that related to mortality in Thailand. Furthermore, the heat stress-related mortality effects are used to assess the heat stress-related mortality for future climate change in Thailand. This part is the important section of the health impact assessment for measuring the heat-related deaths as a result of climate change in the future. The results from this paper will be useful for assessing the implications for population health when climate change makes Thailand hotter.

Chapter 8: Discussion and conclusion: this final chapter presents the overall discussion for the principal findings of health implication in relation to the research objectives and research question. It also discusses the limitations of the study and the validity of the results. It ends up with attention being drawn to the implications for future research about the health impact assessment for heat stress in Thailand.

CHAPTER 2: LITERATURE REVIEW

2.1 Overview

Heat stress has become an important issue in public health and environmental epidemiology. Many researchers have revealed substantial health impacts from heat stress as a direct implication of climate change (Basu and Samet 2002b; Kovats and Hajat 2008; Basu 2009; Kjellstrom 2009b; Kjellstrom and Weaver 2009). This chapter is a detailed review of the relevant literature on heat stress effects on human health and well-being as well as climate change effects on heat stress-related health outcomes. The key themes and unresolved issues of heat stress-related health outcomes are presented. The final section of this chapter is the conclusion highlighting the unanswered issues which become the research questions of this thesis.

2.1.1 Definition of heat stress

The definition of heat stress by American Conference of Industrial Hygienists (ACGIH) is

> *Heat stress is the net (overall) heat burden on the body from the combination of the body heat generated while working, environmental sources (air temperature, humidity, air movement, radiation from the sun or hot surfaces/sources) and clothing requirements* (ACGIH 2008).

Heat stress is one of the physical hazards impacting on human health. Parsons (2003) states that heat stress is a combination of four aspects of thermal environments which include air temperature, radiant heat, humidity, and air movement. During hot weather, the high air temperature and humidity, low wind speed and varying radiation conditions are main factors leading to heat stress, causing discomfort and stress to the human body.

2.1.2 History of heat stress and health

Heat stress and its effects on human health were documented in 1748 by the Baron de Montesquieu who wrote a book entitled "The Spirit of Laws" (Baron de Montesquieu 1748). This wide-ranging work includes a discussion of the relationships between climate and human health. Montesquieu argued that climate is an important causal factor in shaping the general characteristics of people and societies. In particular, he pointed out one impact of heat stress by stating that:

> *There are countries where the excess of heat enervates the body, and renders men so slothful and dispirited that nothing but the fear of chastisement can oblige them to perform any laborious duty: slavery is there more reconcilable to reason* (Baron de Montesquieu 1748, Book XV, Chapter 7, p.240).

He reluctantly accepted that hot weather might provide an argument to justify slavery. In hot country, people feel tired and do not want to perform hard physical work: only punishment can make people work under such undesirable conditions. Montesquieu was not convinced by this argument – he went on to claim that

> *Possibly there is not that climate upon earth where the most laborious services might not with proper encouragement be performed by freemen* (Baron de Montesquieu 1748, Book XV, Chapter 8, p.241).

The reason is that the freeman works with a hope of gain rather than a fear of being punished. Mostesquieu was clearly, and famously, opposed to slavery – nevertheless he is important to our narrative because he accepts a connection between hot weather and human well-being in this context. Beyond physical effects on the body, Montesquieu was perhaps the first to associate heat stress with mental conditions and social norms, for example, the state of slavery. He indicated that heat stress causes people to be inactive and lose enthusiasm. Although Montesquieu's view was not based on empirical data, it provided a new insight on the impact of heat stress.

In the 1800s, studies on the effects of climate on human health began to consider heat stress and its health effects, especially among the military. The historical review by Hollowell (2010) summarises information from studies since the 1880s about heat stress exposure and the potential effects on human health, focusing on the military and colonial services. In 1887, the effect of heat stress on the bodies of soldiers was recorded, particularly heat stroke symptoms (Hunter 1887). In the latter half of the 19th century, there was a clearer picture of heat stress-related health and well-being impacts in the military and occupational settings (Hollowell 2010).

In the early 1900s, the physiological effects of heat stress appeared in many studies and extended to focus on heat tolerance and acclimatisation (Macpherson 1960; Wyndham et al. 1968). A study in Singapore investigated the physiological responses to hot environments and heat acclimatisation in the tropical climate from 1948 to 1953 (Macpherson 1960). This study described that heat tolerance can improve by repeating expose to heat (Macpherson 1960).

Since the 1960s, research has extended to quantify the relationship between meteorological condition and health outcomes as concern about environmental pollution is increasing (Boyd 1960; Ellis 1972; Bull and Morton 1978; Greenberg et al. 1983; Basu and Samet 2002b). The risk factors and vulnerable population of heat stress effects have been investigated (Kilbourne et al. 1982). The heat stress effects on health of workers who are often exposed to heat have been reported, especially among factory and mine workers (Ramsey et al. 1983; MMWR 1984).

One of the main concern of heat stress effects is the excessive mortality and hospital admissions during extreme heat events (Bridger et al. 1976), especially the 1995 Chicago heat wave (Semenza et al. 1996; Semenza et al. 1999) and the 2003 European heat wave (Dear et al. 2005; Kovats and Kristie 2006). In the 2000s, the increase of heat wave events has raised public concern about effects of climate change on human health (Patz et al. 2000; McMichael and Githeko 2001). Many epidemiological studies on health impact assessment of global climate change have provided evidence and analysis approaches to explore the projected heat stress and anticipated health impacts at population level as well as recommendations for future research (Campbell-Lendrum and Woodruff 2007; Patz et al. 2008). The negative impacts of climate change are expected to increase adverse health outcomes in the future as a result of an increase in average temperature and increase the number of hot days and warm nights (Kalkstein 1993; Basu and Samet 2002b; Confalonieri et al. 2007)

Also during the 2000s, Kjellstrom initiated a programme of research focusing on the effects of heat exposure on labour productivity in the hot working environment (Kjellstrom 2000). He raised the important issue of the health of working populations and the reduction of work capacity due to climate change, especially in low and middle income countries (Kjellstrom 2009b).

2.1.3 Physiology of heat stress to human body

Humans suffer from heat stress if their bodies cannot adapt to hot conditions and cannot maintain their normal thermoregulatory system (Bridger 2003). It is important to understand the mechanisms of how the human body responds to heat stress in hot environments. This section describes the mechanisms of thermoregulation inside the body and heat acclimatisation.

Generally, the human body uses thermoregulatory systems to maintain and control heat gain and heat loss from the body (Burton 1934, Parsons 2003). There are two sources of heat stress exposure, external (heat from the environment) and internal (heat from metabolic heat production in the body). Human physiology normally controls the core body temperature at around 37 degrees Celsius (°C) in order to keep body performance and maintain a proper balance between the metabolic heat in body and the environmental heat to which it is exposed (Burton 1934, Parsons 2003).

During excessive heat stress exposure, the underlying mechanisms controlled by the thermoregulatory system are responsible for decreasing body temperature. Those mechanisms include increases in cardiac output and heart rate to deliver blood to the skin surface in order to release the heat out of the body (Wyndham et al. 1968). Also, the body produces sweat to get rid of heat from the skin by evaporation (Sohar 1982).

Parsons (2003) described that the physical methods used by humans for heat loss include radiation, convection, conduction, and evaporation of sweat. Radiation is the outward flow of thermal energy or heat loss from an internal heat to the surrounding environment by electromagnetic waves. Convection is the transfer process of heat from skin surface to environment through movement of surrounding air or water. Conduction is the process of heat transferring between surfaces of body through direct contact to an adjacent cooler surface. Evaporation is the cooling process of sweat droplets at skin surface changing state from liquid to gas (water vapour) suspended in air (Parsons 2003).

However, during hot weather when the air temperature is higher than 35°C, only evaporation of sweat can lower body temperature (Parsons 2003). Evaporation of sweat works less effectively when the relative humidity is higher than 80%. The high vapour content in the environment reduces the sweat evaporation and contributes to increase the body temperature (Parsons 2003). If the relative humidity reaches 100% with the stagnant air condition, the sweat cannot evaporate and the body cooling mechanisms will be limited (Sohar 1982).

2.1.4 Heat acclimatisation

The human body can improve its physiological ability to tolerate heat after repeating exposure to heat stress. This is a process of acclimatisation (Wyndham et al. 1968). For example, on the first few days of heat exposure in summer, the human body responds to heat and shows an increase in body temperature, heart rate and general discomfort (Wyndham et al. 1968). If the body is gradually exposed to heat, heat acclimatisation will improve the thermoregulatory system by increasing sweat rate to get rid of excessive heat (Pandolf 1997; Bridger 2003). After heat acclimatisation, the loss of electrolytes, the blood flow, the heart rate and the body temperature will gradually decrease and become stable (Parsons 2003). Under normal health conditions, a period of heat acclimatisation usually takes about a week and then the body can later adapt to higher temperatures or can make continued exposure to heat stress more acceptable (Parsons 2003).

Human bodies vary in their ability to acclimatise to heat stress (Bridger 2003). People who live in hot and humid countries can tolerate higher temperature than those in non-tropical countries, because they are already acclimatised to the local climate and environment (Ellis 1976). In general, people feel uncomfortable if the air temperature is outside the range of 17 to 31°C (World Health Organization 2010), but the heat tolerance range of some people is narrower than this because they have difficulty acclimatising (Bridger 2003). The ability for heat acclimatisation is limited by high heat exposure, aging, low fitness, overweight, alcoholism, dehydration, sleep deprivation, existing health problems, or using some medications.

At high temperatures, impaired behavioural and physiological responses to heat stress had been reported among the elderly (Ellis 1976), the socially isolated (Pandolf 1997), infants and young children (Sheffield and Landrigan 2011) and obese people (Coris et al. 2004). Smokers and alcohol drinkers are at risk of hyperthermia during hot (Cusack et al. 2011). People who have existing chronic disease, particularly heart or lungs problems, have difficulty in heat acclimatisation (Ellis 1976; Bridger 2003). People who lack sleep and those who return to hot environment after a vacation may not adequately adjust themselves to the hot environment and they are more likely to have heat-related illness due to a lack of acclimatisation (Oechsli and Buechley 1970; Schwartz 2005; Medina-Ramon et al. 2006).

2.2 Heat stress effects on human health and well-being

Several recent studies have summarised the underlying mechanisms and effects of heat stress exposure (Nag et al. 2007; Kovats and Hajat 2008; Basu 2009; Kjellstrom 2009b; Hajat et al. 2010). These sections summarise the literature on previous studies of the heat stress effects on human health and well-being including physical health impacts, mental health impacts, human well-being impacts, occupational health impacts, and heat-related deaths, respectively.

2.2.1 Physical health impacts

The physical health impacts from heat stress are classified into acute and chronic health impacts. Excessive exposure to heat stress can cause acute effects to human health such as heat-related illness or fatal heat stroke (Wyndham 1965). On the other hand, the chronic effects of heat stress can increase risks from other related diseases and injuries (Kjellstrom et al. 2010).

1) Heat-related illnesses

Several studies have investigated the acute effects of heat stress on human health. Early studies reported the high incidence of heat stroke during the Mecca pilgrimage (Hajj) (Weiner and Khogali 1980), among the military and workers (Wyndham 1965; Nag et al. 2007), and people exercising during hot weather (Schrier et al. 1970; Lumlertgul et al. 1992). More recent studies about the acute health impacts of heat exposure concern the effects of climate change, especially heat wave events (Kovats and Hajat 2008; Robine et al. 2008; Knowlton et al. 2009; Nitschke et al. 2011; Wang et al. 2011b).

The acute effects of heat stress occur when the body cannot maintain the core temperature or cannot acclimatise to heat stress (Parsons 2003). These acute effects are the heat-related illness which can be categorised according to the severity of symptom from heat rash, heat cramps, heat syncope and heat exhaustion, to the serious heat stroke (Bouchama and Knochel 2002).

Heat rash or prickly heat is likely to occur in hot and humid environments where sweat is unable to evaporate and the skin continuously remains wet (OSHA 2005). The sweat ducts become plugged, and then a skin rash soon appears. Heat rash is not life-threatening. When the rash is extensive, it may itch or hurt and prickly heat can be very uncomfortable (OSHA 2005).

Heat cramps are sudden and painful contraction of the muscles, especially part of the arms, legs, or abdomen (Parsons 2009). Heat cramps occur among those who sweat a lot during hot weather and drink a large quantity of water, but do not sufficiently replace the body's electrolytes lost from blood and muscle tissues (OSHA 2005). Drinking of a large quantity of water without adequate salt tends to dilute the body's fluids and results in a low sodium state in the muscles. As a result, the low salt level in the muscles causes cramps. However, it is not life-threatening (OSHA 2005).

Heat syncope or fainting occurs due to lack of acclimatisation (Parsons 2003). It can happen during the first few days of heat stress exposure, especially when the air temperature rises suddenly. The body tries to release the excessive internal heat by increasing blood flow to the skin rather than to the heart or other internal organs (Parsons 2003). As a result, a person who has inadequate heat acclimatisation can faint due to the decreased blood and oxygen supply to the brain (Parsons 2009).

Heat exhaustion is less severe than heat stroke (Parsons 2009). If the core body temperature exceeds 38°C over several hours due to prolonged heat stress exposure and dehydration, heat exhaustion will occur and can lead quickly to heat stroke (Ramsey 1995). Heat exhaustion is caused by water depletion or loss of large amount of fluid by sweating, or excessive loss of important electrolytes (Cho and Lee 1978). A person suffering from heat exhaustion still sweats but experiences severe weakness, fatigue, dizziness, nausea, headache, discomfort and dehydration with only minimally altered mental status (Bouchama and Knochel 2002).

Heat stroke is the most serious problem of heat-related illness. It occurs when the body's thermoregulatory mechanisms are overwhelmed by heat stress, especially when the core temperature exceeds 40°C, and sweating becomes inadequate or stops (Bouchama and Knochel 2002; Parsons 2009). When the core body temperature rises, blood flow generally shifts from the vital organs to the body's skin to release heat. If the body cannot control the core temperature and too much blood is diverted, it will result in hyperthermia and central nervous system dysfunction (Bouchama and Knochel 2002). Victims of heat stroke are mentally confused and unconscious, and death can occur within hours (Lumlertgul et al. 1992; Bouchama and Knochel 2002). The underlying factors of fatal heat stroke are described in the studies among the

South African mine workers (Wyndham 1965) or crop workers in the United States (MMWR 2008).

2) Heat stress increases risks from other related diseases and injuries

Many diseases are associated with climate variation or extreme hot conditions (Patz et al. 2005). The immediate health impacts of heat stress may not be noticed at the time of high heat exposure but may influence on chronic disease occurrence and impact on pre-existing illness (Kjellstrom 2009a; Kjellstrom et al. 2010). The accumulated effects of heat stress can exacerbate existing diseases or chronic disorders such as cardiovascular or respiratory illnesses, kidney disease (McMichael and Githeko 2001; McMichael et al. 2003; Riedel 2004; Patz et al. 2005; Kjellstrom et al. 2010).

Prolonged heat stress exposure can affect cardiovascular and respiratory systems because the body core temperature increased, the blood flow shifts away from the vital organs to the skin surface to cool the body (Parsons 2003). If the body has inadequate heat acclimatisation and too much blood does not return to those core organs, it will increase stress on the heart and lungs (Kovats and Hajat 2008). Heat stress can add strain to the body system such as increased platelet, red blood cell count and plasma viscosity; in severe situations this can lead to dehydration and hypertension (Wyndham et al. 1968). Moreover, increases in heart rate and respiratory volume to release heat from the body also increase the daily intake of some environmental hazards such as air pollutants and allergenic pollens (Kjellstrom 2009a).

Many studies have shown that heat stress is associated with hospital admission or deaths with cardiovascular, cerebrovascular and respiratory diseases in Australia (Loughnan et al. 2010; Nitschke et al. 2011; Wang et al. 2011b), Europe (Robine et al. 2008), the United States (Knowlton et al. 2009) and China (Huang et al. 2010; Guo et al. 2011; Liu et al. 2011a). However, a study in Denmark reported that increasing heat stress is associated with an increase in hospital admissions for respiratory diseases, but a decrease for cardiovascular diseases (Wichmann et al. 2011).

Heat stress can increase the risk of kidney disease due to dehydration (Schrier et al. 1970). During summer or hot weather, a high rate of evaporation by sweating to release heat from the body can result in loss of body water and electrolytes especially sodium and chloride (Parsons 2003). This water and sodium depletion results in loss of extracellular fluid volume, which can place acute or chronic stress on kidney function and ultimately lead to kidney disease (Schrier et al. 1970). Kidney disease is categorised into acute kidney failure (sudden loss of kidney function from severe dehydration) and chronic kidney failure (slow, gradual loss of kidney function). Slow loss of kidney function is exacerbated by diabetes, hypertension, and blockage from kidney stones (Brikowski et al. 2008). Heat waves and related dehydration are associated with both acute and chronic kidney failure (Semenza et al. 1999; Hansen et al. 2008b; Knowlton et al. 2009; Cervellin et al. 2011; Fakheri and Goldfarb 2011). As a result, the increase of kidney disease is an outcome of climate change (Kjellstrom et al. 2010).

Moreover, people fatigued from heat stress are more susceptible to accident and injury. The relationship between heat stress and injury occurrence had been reported many times over the last four decades (Cho and Lee 1978; Ramsey et al. 1983; Enander and Hygge 1990; Fogleman et al. 2005; Morabito et al. 2006). Excessive heat exposure can increase the risk of injury. This may be due to fainting, confusion, poor concentration, and psychological distress (Hancock 1981, Hancock and Warm 1989).

2.2.2 Mental health impacts

Heat stress can pose a salient risk to mental health. Hansen et al. (2008a) observed the heat-stress related mental health outcomes during heat waves in 1993 and 2006 in Australia. They reported an increase in the number of hospital admissions with dementia, mental and mood disorders during the heat waves (Hansen et al. 2008a).

Increasing heat stress is associated with higher rates of aggressive behaviour and suicide (Anderson et al. 2000; Anderson 2001). Page et al. (2007) observed that an increase in heat stress was associated with an increase in suicide risk during heat wave in England and Wales. Moreover, Berry et al. (2010) illustrated that the increasing heat stress as a result of climate change can cause psychological distress among workers due to a reduction in work production and a disruption of daily activity.

2.2.3 Human well-being impacts

Heat stress can affect human well-being by disrupting time spent on personal activities including work, travel, sleep, and leisure time (Kjellstrom 2009b). People find it difficult to work and feel uncomfortable when performing their daily activities under heat stress because of tiredness or psychological strain from exhaustion (Wyndham 1969). Also, a person who suffers from heat stress, especially a manual worker, is more likely to have low coordination, alertness, endurance and vigilance to conduct their work (Mathee et al. 2010). As a result, heat stress causes disruption to well-being by reduced physical and work performance (Hancock and Vasmatzidis 1998; Hancock et al. 2007), and has negative influence on life satisfaction and quality of life (Kjellstrom 2009b).

2.2.4 Occupational health impacts

Recently, studies of heat stress from climate change have drawn attention to adverse health effects among workers (Kjellstrom 2000; Kjellstrom 2009b). The international program "High Occupational Temperature Health and Productivity Suppression (HOTHAPS)" has been developed and conducted many studies focusing on the effects of heat exposure on working people (Kjellstrom et al. 2009a). Currently, these research projects have extended their studies to many areas, especially tropical developing countries (Kjellstrom 2009b; Kjellstrom et al. 2009a; Ingole et al. 2012).

Ingole (2012) found an association between heat stress and mortality among people aged from 20 to 50 years old in India, a hot and humid country. Persons in this age group are more likely to be in the workforce and are often exposed to heat during work (Kjellstrom et al. 2009b). The working population who spend most of their time in a hot environment are vulnerable to heat stress especially those who carry out heavy work which produces internal heat (Parsons 2003; Kjellstrom et al. 2009a). People with low incomes who are doing heavy labour outdoors, such as poor farmers or labourers, are at the greatest risk of heat stress effects (Kjellstrom et al. 2009b). These workers do demanding jobs during hot days and don't have heat protection, increasing the risk of clinical health effects and poor working performance (Kjellstrom and Weaver 2009). Also, they may keep working during the heat in order to complete work tasks to get paid, putting their heat exposure over the safe limit (Kjellstrom 2000; Kjellstrom et al. 2009a).

Physically active workers especially those who work outdoors are more likely to have health impacts from heat stress effects even if they are fit and healthy (Kjellstrom et al. 2009a). These may result from a lack of awareness that they are becoming ill from high temperature; therefore they ignore their dehydration and do not take action to reduce heat exposure. If workers have insufficient water intake and sweat substantially, they will increase the loss of their body fluid volume and become dehydrated which can create adverse health impacts (such as heat stroke, heat-related illness or kidney disease) (Bridger 2003). Moreover, they can get exhausted from heat stress and perform their works disregarding their safety protection. Consequently, heat stress can increase unsafe working conditions and also occupational injuries (Ramsey et al. 1983; Mathee et al. 2010).

For mental health impacts on workers, if they are exposed to excessive heat and their body cannot cool down, they could experience severe psychological distress caused by heat exhaustion (Wyndham 1965; Wyndham 1969; Hancock 1981). Moreover, workers who often work under heat stress have a potential to develop long-term mental health problems such as chronic depression or anxiety disorders (Hansen et al. 2008a). Hancock and Vasmatzidis (2003) indicated that workers face a high risk of heat stress effects and a reduced performance efficiency if they perform difficult cognitive tasks under prolonged heat exposure beyond the heat safe limits.

Working in the hot environment not only has negative impact on health, but also affects work capacity (Kjellstrom et al. 2009c). Many studies have shown that heat stress has significant impacts on work capacity and productivity (Hancock and Vasmatzidis 1998; Kjellstrom 2000; Bridger 2003; Hancock and Vasmatzidis 2003; Parsons 2003). For example, Wyndham (1969) and Mathee et al. (2010) observed that

34

outdoor workers who worked in summer in the South Africa had to slow down their work during heat, or rest more often to cool down their bodies. For this reason, workers who take more breaks or work slower because of heat stress will decrease their working hours and reduce their work performance and productivity (Wyndham 1965; Kjellstrom 2000; Kjellstrom et al. 2009b).

A study by Kjellstrom et al (2009c) quantifies the impacts of climate change on workplace heat stress and on work productivity at global and regional level for many regions. The reduction in working hours and productivity as a result of heat stress from climate change in the future will affect well-being of workers by reducing their income and decreasing their life satisfaction (Kjellstrom et al. 2009b).

2.2.5 Heat stress-related deaths

A number of studies show that high temperatures during heat waves are associated with marked short-term increases in mortality (Bridger et al. 1976; Martens 1998; Patz et al. 2000; Basu and Samet 2002b; Confalonieri et al. 2007).

In the United States, the severe heat wave in July 1995 caused at least 700 excess deaths in Chicago with the daily maximum temperature ranging from 34-40°C (MMWR 1995). In July 2006, the number of deaths occurring during a heat wave in California were 665 excess deaths compared with mortality during the non-heatwave period in June and August 2006 (Hoshiko et al. 2010).

In Europe, Robine et al. (2008) identified that more than 70,000 additional deaths were recorded in 16 countries during the heat waves in summer 2003 compared to the baseline mortality during the non-heatwave period of 1998-2002. One of the most severely affected countries was France with over 15,000 deaths from this extreme event (Kovats and Kristie 2006). Furthermore, France faced another severe heat wave in 2006, leading to over 2,000 excess deaths (Fouillet et al. 2008).

In Australia, the number of deaths increased during the heat wave in February 2004 with excess of 75 non-external deaths and 45 cardiovascular deaths in Brisbane (Tong et al. 2010). During the heat wave in January 2009, the three consecutive days of maximum temperatures above 43°C were recorded with 374 excess deaths in Victoria compared to a mean of mortality for the previous five years (Victorian Government Department of Human Services 2009). McMichael et al. (2003) estimated that each year in Australian capital cities, the excess deaths of 1,100 people who aged over 65 years were associated with high temperatures.

In China, the daily maximum temperature fluctuation in Shanghai during the heat wave in August 1998 showed 258 excess deaths compared with the baseline number of deaths from June to September (Huang et al. 2010). In India, the heat waves were estimated to cause 1,658 heat-related deaths in March 1998 and 1,539 deaths in 2003 (Akhtar 2007).

Those previous studies focused on the effects of heat waves on mortality by estimating the excess death or a proportion of the additional mortality during heat wave compared with baseline mortality during the period without a heat wave (Fouillet et al. 2008; Robine et al. 2008; Hoshiko et al. 2010). Moreover, many studies explored daily changes in the number of deaths associated with the temperature variation during hot or cold seasons, rather than heat waves (Basu and Samet 2002b). For example studies in England and Wales showed strongly significant associations between temperatures during winter and some specific causes of death: for example, myocardial infarction, strokes and pneumonia (Bull and Morton 1978), as well as cerebrovascular diseases (Haberman et al. 1981).

2.3 Risk factors for heat stress effects on health and well-being

Many studies identified the population at high risks of heat stress by considering the risk factors that can increase the likelihood of heat exposure or affect heat stress-related health outcomes (Wyndham 1965; Bridger et al. 1976; Katsouyanni K et al. 1993; Kenney and Munce 2003; O'Neill et al. 2005; Bouchama et al. 2007; Kovats and Hajat 2008; Schifano et al. 2009). The risk factors include individual risk factors (such as age, existing chronic illness, heavy physical activity and insufficient heat protection) and socioeconomic factors (such as poverty, social isolation, housing condition, air conditioning, urban residents and air pollution).

2.3.1 Individual risk factors

During summer or high environmental temperature, many people are exposed to excessive heat even higher than their body core temperature range. The most vulnerable group are the elderly (Kenney and Munce 2003) and infants (Bridger et al. 1976). A study in Italy by Schifano et al. (2009) reported that the excess mortality was highest among elderly people with existing chronic disease during the summers of 2005-2007. This may be due to low physical fitness level and impaired physiological response to heat stress.

People who have existing health problems or take certain medications are at risk of heat stress. Some medicines can inhibit sweating, reduce heat elimination and reduce people's physiological adaptation to heat (Kwok and Chan 2005; Cusack et al. 2011). Diuretic drugs can increase the level of dehydration due to loss of fluids and electrolytes from the body (Coris et al. 2004). Antidepressants, antipsychotics, and antihistamines can reduce the capacity of central nervous system to control body temperature (Bark 1998; Kaiser et al. 2001; Coris et al. 2004; Kwok and Chan 2005).

Among healthy people who undertake heavy physical activities during hot conditions, heat is generated inside the body and also gained from the hot environment (Parsons 2003). These people are at risk of heat stress effects because of inadequate hydration or inappropriate clothing (Greenberg et al. 1983). Several studies already presented the heat stress effects on health among those who are doing exercise (Coris et al. 2004), males in military service (Yaglou and Minard 1957), workers in heavy labour work (Mathee et al. 2010; Kjellstrom and Crowe 2011) such as mine workers (Wyndham 1965) and agricultural workers (MMWR 2008).

2.3.2 Socioeconomic factors

There is a wide array of socioeconomic factors that can increase the vulnerability to heat stress exposure (Hajat et al. 2005; Bell et al. 2008; Hajat et al. 2010). These socioeconomic factors include poverty, social isolation, poor housing conditions or living in urban area (Bouchama et al. 2007; Kovats and Hajat 2008).

Poor urban populations living in low and middle income countries are of particular concern (Basu and Samet 2002a). There are many poor urban populations residing in informal settlements or slums where there is a high-density of poor housing facilities, or no air conditioning (Confalonieri et al. 2007). Semenza et al. (1996) and Kaiser et al. (2007) noted that the poor urban populations and those with fewer social connections were at higher risk of death during the 1995 Chicago heat wave. During hot weather, people who lack access to essential facilities (such as adequate clean water, or air conditioning) are more likely to have adverse health effects from heat stress (O'Neill et al. 2005).

Using air conditioning is one of the methods that reduces heat stress exposure; it helps maintain a comfortable condition, especially in homes, buildings, or at working place (Koppe et al. 2004). A few studies have indicated that air conditioning can prevent heat stroke and heat-related illness during heat waves in the United States (Semenza et al. 1996). The usage of air-conditioners can also reduce the heat stress effects on morbidity outcomes, such as hospital admissions for multiple diseases including respiratory disease, cardiovascular diseases, ischemic stroke, heat stroke, dehydration, diabetes, and acute renal failure in California (Ostro et al. 2010).

However, the increased use of air conditioning is an important factor contributing to increased outdoor temperature, especially in urban areas (Wilby 2003). The increasing use of air conditioning increases energy consumption and can lead to increased greenhouse gas emissions from fuel combustion in energy production processes (Ostro et al. 2010). Moreover, power blackouts often occur during periods of high energy demands in summer or heat wave events, so people who rely on air conditioning in their home, office and elsewhere can be at risk of heat stress effects

(Bridger et al. 1976). For example, office workers in a building with air conditioning may have low ability to acclimatise to outdoor hot environment and are at high risk of heat stress effects. Other options for effective heat protection are building designs such as shading of the building to reduce the solar radiation impacts, increasing green spaces, or increasing natural ventilation in the building (Koppe et al. 2004). The building design with heat protection is important, especially the buildings in urban areas.

Urban climate during hot weather can increase the risk of heat stress effects. The urban climate is local climate being modified by interactions between local air temperature and urban heat-island effect. The concrete buildings or paved roads in urban areas absorb and re-radiate the heat and cause high temperature in city areas (Oke 1973). The urban population living in dense built-up areas are exposed to heat stress at a higher level than rural areas (Clarke 1972; Oke 1973; Kovats and Hajat 2008). The air temperatures in high-density urban areas are generally up to $3°C$ warmer than in surrounding areas (Riedel 2004). Moreover, the urban heat island effect is likely to increase in the future as a result of rapidly increasing urban population (McMichael et al. 2003).

It should be noted that a combined exposure to heat stress and air pollution has possible synergistic effects on health (Katsouyanni K et al. 1993). Air quality during periods of severe heat is likely to have a high level of air pollutions such as ozone (O_3) (Bernard et al. 2001; Ren et al. 2009). The high temperatures and solar radiation can accelerate photochemical reactions which contribute to the rapid formation of O_3 (Bernard et al. 2001). Studies on heat-related deaths found that the combined exposure to high temperatures and air pollutants such as O_3, nitrogen dioxide (NO_2), and particulate matter with diameter under 10 microns (PM_{10}) appears to be a critical risk factor for cardiovascular mortality (Ren et al. 2008; Ren et al. 2009).

The high heat exposure during heat waves showed larger effects on mortality when O_3 levels were high (Dear et al. 2005). Moreover, a study in 11 cities in the Eastern United States reported that combined effect of heat stress with the urban heat-island effect and air pollution was greater than the simple additive effects of these two stresses (Curriero et al. 2002).

2.4 Epidemiological studies for heat stress-related health outcomes

This section presents the study designs and findings of the heat stress-related health outcomes from previous epidemiological studies in order to justify and support the work in this thesis. Many epidemiological studies explored heat-related deaths at the population level as the weather and mortality data are available (Bouchama et al. 2007; Kovats and Hajat 2008; Basu 2009). Those existing studies investigated the relationship between heat stress and mortality by using a variety of heat exposure indicators and statistical modelling techniques.

2.4.1 Heat exposure indicators

Many epidemiological studies explored the heat stress-related health outcomes by using available mortality and meteorological data. The meteorological data are usually obtained from local weather stations and represent the heat stress exposure of the population in and nearby that area. Many studies have used direct measurement of weather variables. The simply daily maximum, minimum and mean temperatures are readily available from monitoring stations, easy to understand and applicable for the studies of daily temperature and health relationship (Epstein and Moran 2006). Alternatively, humidity, radiant heat or wind speed have been combined with the air temperature to present heat stress exposure based on heat physiology mechanisms (Epstein and Moran 2006). The apparent temperature, heat index, humidex and wet-bulb globe temperature are selected as the examples of heat exposure indicators in this section.

Apparent Temperature is a combination of humidity and air temperature representing physical discomfort (Steadman 1984). The association between daily apparent temperature and health outcomes was reported in many studies. For example, the association between daily mean apparent temperature and total mortality was reported from Seoul (1991-2006), Beijing (1998-2000), Tokyo (1972-1994) and Taipei (1994-2003) with the threshold apparent temperature ranging from 25.2 to 33.5°C (Chung et al. 2009). However, Kinny et al. (2008) suggested that the formula of apparent temperature appears to be a problem because it can increase due to low temperature and high humidity, while actually the apparent temperature is expected to increase only in the hot weather (Kinney et al. 2008).

Heat Index is a combination of heat and humidity conditions. The United States National Oceanic and Atmospheric Administration use the heat index to forecast and to provide heat warnings to the public of the United States (National Weather Service 2012). A study by Metzger et al. reported a linear association between the same-day maximum heat index and mortality during 1997 and 2006 in New York City. They reported that the associations between mortality and maximum heat index values for the one, two, or three days prior were non-linear, with a sharp increase in predicted mortality for heat index values between 35 and 38°C (Metzger et al. 2009).

Humidex is an equivalent index for the combined effects of relative humidity and temperature. The weather service of Environment Canada uses the humidex to inform public when conditions of heat and humidity are potentially uncomfortable (Canadian Centre for Occupational Health and Safety 2008). For example, a study by Jackson et al. (2010) found a relationship between the daily maximum humidex and mortality in the elderly (ages 65 and above) in Washington State during 1980 and 2006.

Wet-bulb globe temperature (WBGT) is widely used in the international and national occupational health guidelines to measure workplace heat stress conditions (Lemke and Kjellstrom 2012). It is a combined index of the four fundamental weather variables determining human exposure including air temperature, humidity, air movement and radiant heat (Yaglou and Minard 1957). The WBGT index had been developed and validated by studies since the 1950s (Yaglou and Minard 1957; Bernard and Pourmoghani 1999; Liljegren et al. 2008). Lemke and Kjellstrom (2012) concluded that the WBGT formula of Liljegren et al. (2008) is the best for WBGT outdoors while the formula of Bernard and Pourmoghani (1999) is suitable to calculate the WBGT indoors by assuming no heat radiation. The findings from the

41

WBGT are easy to interpret for exposure-response relationship, so it is widely used as the heat exposure indicator to investigate its association with health outcomes or work performance (Wyndham 1965; Ayyappan et al. 2009; Mathee et al. 2010).

Furthermore, some studies use the heat exposure indicators based on calculations of meteorological data and physiological variables such as metabolic rate, or clothing depending on their research purposes (Epstein and Moran 2006). These complex heat exposure indicators can reflect heat removal capacities of humans; an example is the Universal Thermal Climate Index (UTCI) (Parsons 2003; Epstein and Moran 2006).

Universal Thermal Climate Index (UTCI) is recently developed to represent the human physiological response to the heat in the environment. It is based on physiological modelling of human thermoregulation (Fiala D et al. 2001). UTCI is sensitive to changes in ambient temperature, solar radiation, humidity and especially wind speed (Blazejczyk et al. 2012). UTCI has been used in some studies, for example, a study about thermal comfort under the current situation and future climate change in Hong Kong (Cheung and Hart 2012).

Heat exposure indicators mentioned above are some of the heat exposure indexes that have been developed and used in many studies. A study by Epstein and Moran (2006) reviews the heat stress exposure indicators over 40 indexes that have been developed since the 19th century. Those indicators attempt to represent the heat stress exposure by combining the physiological and environmental variables related to heat stress. However, none of the existing heat exposure indicators has been accepted as a universal index (Epstein and Moran 2006).

Currently, the most often used index during the last decades is the WBGT index (Epstein and Moran 2006). WBGT is adopted as an international standard for occupational heat exposure (ISO 1989) and is also used in the recommendations from the American Conference of Governmental Industrial Hygienists as a criterion for occupational heat stress (ACGIH 2008). The standard recommends a limited hour of work and a rest time at different WBGT levels which aims to protect health of workers who are exposed to heat at work (ISO 1989) .

2.4.2 Methods for assessing heat stress-related health outcomes

Significant associations between heat stress and health outcomes have been reported in several epidemiological studies (Semenza et al. 1996; Kalkstein and Greene 1997). Those studies have identified these associations by using different heat stress variables or statistical modellings. A number of studies consider deaths above the threshold temperature (McMichael et al. 2008; Armstrong et al. 2011), deaths at particular percentile of temperature (Medina-Ramon et al. 2006) or taking into account of the short-term effects and harvesting effects (Braga et al. 2001; Hajat et al. 2005). Also, some studies explored the relationship between mortality and temperatures alone or effect modification by certain factors such as high humidity, wind speed, air pressure and cloud cover, as well as the possible synergistic effects from air pollution (Basu and Samet 2002b; Ren et al. 2008; Hajat et al. 2010).

3) Statistical modelling for heat-related deaths

Understanding the strengths and weaknesses of various types of studies will help determine the suitable approach for identifying the association between heat stress and mortality in this thesis. This section summarises the statistical approaches often used in the studies on heat-related deaths including time-series and case-crossover studies.

1.1)   Time-series design and statistical modelling

In environmental epidemiology studies, the time-series approach is a well-known study design that documents the association between temperature and mortality by using a wide range of modelling techniques. The typical time-series regression is suitable for estimating the effects of heat stress exposure over a period of time from one day to several days by comparing daily counts of deaths as an outcome variable with the temperature on the same day or over the last few days (or lagged days) (Gasparrini and Armstrong 2010).

This time-series design of heat-related deaths aims to estimate the change in the number of deaths associated with temperature, controlling for potential confounders such as long-term trend, season, air pollution, or epidemics of influenza (Gasparrini and Armstrong 2010). Similar to the study methods for air pollution epidemiology, the time-series approach is often used for quantifying an association between air pollution and daily death. However, there are some differences between the time-series study for assessing the health impacts from air temperature and the heat impacts from air pollution. For example, temperature-related mortality has a non-linear relationship such as a U- or V-shape (Gasparrini and Armstrong 2010), while the air pollution-related mortality typically has a linear association (Dominici 2004).

The statistical modelling techniques for time-series studies have been developed from simple linear regression methods to more sophisticated modelling approaches. The daily counts of deaths can be assumed to be a Poisson distribution thus the simple methods of Poisson regression models can filter out the long-term trend (such as population growth or change and technology change) and seasonal variation in daily health outcomes and weather variation (Gasparrini and Armstrong 2010).

The techniques for conducting non-linear regression analysis in time-series studies such as generalised linear model (GLM), generalised additive model (GAM) or generalised estimating equation (GEE) are commonly used in the recent time-series analyses (Gasparrini and Armstrong 2010). These three models allow users to adjust for linear or non-linear terms of daily temperature, over-dispersion or confounding effects of trends and seasonality.

Some studies used the GLM with parametric regression splines such as natural and cubic splines. A single spline function of time has been used to produce an irregular seasonal trend which is believed to control additional confounding effects operating at medium timescales (Piver et al. 1999; Vaneckova et al. 2008; Chung et al. 2009; Gasparrini and Armstrong 2010)

The GAM extensively is used for exploring the short-term effects of heat stress on mortality (Curriero et al. 2003; Dominici 2004; El-Zein and Tewtel-Salem 2005). The

GAM is more flexible than GLM because GAM can be used to explore many nonparametric relationships simultaneously by using nonparametric smoothing such as Loess smoothing technique adjusting for temperature or potential confounders such as season, effects of the day of week, other weather variables and air pollution variables that vary on a daily basis. The dependent variable in GAM is the natural logarithm of the expected number of deaths, and the regression coefficients are the natural logarithms of the rate ratio. However, GAM has a collinearity problem for non-linear functions (Dominici et al. 2002; Ramsay et al. 2003) as well as the difficulty in specifying the type of smoother and the number of degrees of freedom to adjust for changes overtime (Carracedo-Martinez et al. 2010). Also, the nonparametric smoothing in GAM could lead to biased estimates and to underestimate the true variance (Dominici et al. 2002).

The GEE is an extended approach from GLM (Baccini et al. 2008). The GEE has been used in the analysis of health effects from air pollution by Schwartz and Dockery (1992). Some recent studies used GEE to investigate the health effects from heat waves (Hajat et al. 2006; Fouillet et al. 2007; Williams et al. 2012). For example, a study by Baccini et al. (2008) used the GEE approach to explore the exposure-response curves of heat-related deaths in 15 European cities. They stated that GEE is suitable for longitudinal data analysis when mortality is assumed to be independent of different summer periods, while the deaths in the same summer season are assumed to be correlated (Baccini et al. 2008).

1.2)   *Case-crossover design and statistical modelling*

A case-crossover design has been recently conducted to evaluate the acute effects of temperature on health outcomes (Barnett 2007). It is adapted from a case-control design to study the effects of transient exposure on the occurrence of acute events (Maclure 1991). For example, only deaths (cases) during heat wave are analysed by comparing the heat exposure on the day of death with the exposures of same person in nearby days. This matched sets of exposure in the same person are called "reference windows" (Janes et al. 2005a).

The case-crossover design is suited for exploring the temperature-related deaths when individual-level mortality records data are available. Date record of person death is considered as a case day comparing with nearby days (control days) in order to represent the exposure distribution during the time periods when that person is alive (Carracedo-Martinez et al. 2010). There are many different types of case-crossover designs depending on the selection of control days. Unidirectional design, bidirectional designs (and their subtypes) and up to time-stratified case-crossover designs have been developed respectively (Carracedo-Martinez et al. 2010).

First, the unidirectional design is the initial case-crossover design. This design selects one or more control days before the case day (Mittleman et al. 1995). However, the unidirectional design does not control for the trends over time of exposure variables or health outcomes, and so can be subject to bias (Greenland 1996; Greenland 2001). Therefore, if there is no trend in exposures, a unidirectional design can be used by selecting control days prior to the case day.

The bidirectional designs have been developed to reduce the bias of time trends in exposure which there are three different subtypes in the choice of control periods (Carracedo-Martinez et al. 2010). The different types in bidirectional case-crossover designs include the full-stratum case–crossover (Navidi 1998), symmetric case–crossover (Bateson and Schwartz 1999) and semi-symmetric case–crossover design (Navidi and Weinhandl 2002). First, the full-stratum bidirectional case–crossover is designed to choose the control days from all exposure periods in the time series before and after the case days (Navidi 1998). This full-stratum bidirectional design controls time trends in exposure, but does not control seasonal patterns in exposure or health outcomes (Bateson and Schwartz 1999).

Second, the symmetrical bidirectional case–crossover design takes two control days, one before and one after the case day and equally far from the case day (Bateson and Schwartz 1999). This method can control seasonal trends which occur in the above design. However, there is the potential for selection bias because the cases at the beginning or the end of the data series have fewer control days for matching (Bateson and Schwartz 2001). Navidi and Weinhandl (2002) noted that the symmetric case–

crossover design is biased by time trends of exposure. For example, a study by Liu et al. (2011b) used the symmetrical bidirectional case-crossover design to study effects of heat waves on daily death counts in Beijing, China by selecting the seventh day before and after death as its own self-control between 1 January 1999 and 30 June 2000. They found a significant increase in respiratory mortality during the heat wave with the highest impacts among females aged older than 65 years (Liu et al. 2011b).

Third, the semi-symmetric case–crossover design selects a control day only before or after the case day at random (Navidi and Weinhandl 2002). This design can control the long-term and seasonal trends the same as the symmetric bidirectional design. Nevertheless, the semisymmetric bidirectional design selects only one control day at a fixed interval, so the estimates can be biased (Levy et al. 2001).

However, the previous case-crossover designs have problem as a result of inappropriate selection for the control days in non-disjointed strata, this bias called the "overlapping bias" (Austin et al. 1989). In order to reduce the bias that could appear in above designs, the time-stratified case–crossover design was developed (Levy et al. 2001). Janes et al. (2005b) demonstrated that the time-stratified design can avoid the overlapping bias by selecting one or several control days falling within the same time stratum when the case events occur.

For example, the control days can be matching on the same day of the week as the case within the same month to create partitions with three or four control days for each case. This stratified by month and by day of the week gives the same maximum distance between case and control. This method can avoid autocorrelation problem and control potential confounders such as day of the week by adding to the model as indicator variables (Carracedo-Martinez et al. 2010).

Advantages of the case-crossover design include that it can eliminate the effects of potential confounders by matching methods, and can examine whether the events are associated with a particular exposure (Lu and Zeger 2007; Darrow 2010). Using matched data and comparison within the same person can control confounding effectively. This study design automatically adjusts for personal by factors such as age, socioeconomic status, personal smoking or dietary habits, as they remain constant for each person during case and control periods (Maclure 1991; Navidi 1998). Moreover, it can reduce bias from selection and misclassification of exposure, overmatching. Also, it can adjust for time-trends and seasonal variation (Navidi 1998; Basu and Malig 2010). Regarding the effects of a long- and short-term trend of seasonality in daily data, the control days should be selected close to the case day (Bateson and Schwartz 2001; Carracedo-Martinez et al. 2010).

The measure of association from a case-crossover study can be shown by odds ratio (OR) or relative risk (RR) and 95% confidence interval (95% CI) (Jaakkola 2003). Typically, the OR is estimated by using conditional logistic regressions or stratified Cox proportional hazards models (Wang et al. 2011a). The conditional logistic regressions are often used to estimate adjusted ORs by dividing the number of cases exposed during the case day by those exposed during the control days.

Basu et al. (2010) identified the association between apparent temperature and preterm delivery by using a time-stratified case-crossover analysis in California during the summer months from 1999 to 2006. The control days were selected at lag six of apparent temperature exposure. They found the association between preterm deaths and the weekly average apparent temperature (Basu et al. 2010).

Also, Basu et al. (2005) used the time-stratified case-crossover design to explore the association between temperature and cardio-respiratory mortality among the elderly population in the United States. Furthermore, they compared results from the case-crossover design to the time-series analyses. The results showed that the case-crossover design and the time-series analyses are comparable as they provided consistent findings in this study (Basu et al. 2005). The similar result from the case-crossover design and the time-series log-linear model without over-dispersion was also reported in a study by Lepeule et al. (2006).

However, bias in the estimation of health effects by using the time-stratified case-crossover design can occur when the health outcomes and exposure have a trend (Lu et al. 2008). For example, the time-stratified case-crossover design cannot capture the smoothness of daily death under the seasonal trends or day of week effects (Lu et al. 2008). Lu et al. (2008) suggested that a future study using the time-stratified case-crossover design should do the pre-model checking for the time trends to make sure whether they are constant during case and control periods

4) Threshold temperature and shape of association

The outcomes from the above quantitative studies of heat mortality relationship commonly reported a regression coefficient, relative risk from time-series analysis, odds ratio from case-crossover design, or percent change in deaths (Basu 2009). These results can show the magnitude of the heat stress effects when the temperature increases a certain level. In addition, studies on the relationship between heat stress and mortality should involve the complexity of heat exposure and body mechanism through an investigation of the dose-response shape of heat and mortality and an exploration of the temperature threshold.

The threshold temperature is defined as a temperature with no or minimum effect on mortality. It is commonly used to estimate the health effects from exposure to high or low temperature (Ballester et al. 1997; Keatinge et al. 2000; Braga et al. 2002; Curriero et al. 2002; McMichael et al. 2008; Chung et al. 2009). If the threshold temperature exists along with the exposure-response relationship, it will present a non-linear association between temperature and health outcomes as a U-, V- or J-shaped relationship (Basu 2009). The relationship between temperature and mortality in a U- or V-shape presents an increase in death during hot weather as well as cold weather with the lowest number of deaths at bottom of the U-shape (Kunst et al. 1993; Martens 1998). Some studies described the relationship between daily mortality and daily temperature as in reverse J-shaped pattern (Liu et al. 2011a). Where the trough of the J-shape represents the comfort zone and the short arm of the J-shape represents the steeper slope of mortality increase with rising temperature above this comfort zone. The long arm of the J-shape shows the increase in mortality at colder temperatures below that comfort zone (McMichael et al. 2006).

A few studies have reported that cities with warmer climates have higher threshold temperatures than cooler cities (Gosling et al. 2007; Chung et al. 2009). These findings confirmed that the threshold temperatures vary by geography location, weather condition and population group. Consequently, the estimation of heat-related death should take into account regional, seasonal and demographical differences (Kim et al. 2006; Chung et al. 2009).

5) Lagged effect of heat exposure

The risk of mortality from heat stress exposure can occur on the current day and also persist to several days later (Anderson and Bell 2009). The distribution of cumulative effects of heat stress exposure over days or weeks after exposure has been addressed in many time-series studies.

Some studies applied the distributed lag models (DLMs) to create the lag structure of exposure-respond relationships (Armstrong 2006; Rocklov and Forsberg 2008). This distributed lag model is suitable to estimate the heat stress effects particularly during heat waves periods as it allows the linear effect of single heat exposure to be distributed over those period of time (Rocklov and Forsberg 2010). Recently, the distributed lag models have been developed from simple distributed lag models to distributed lag non-linear models (DLNMs) (Gasparrini and Armstrong 2010). The DLNMs are flexible to study the delayed effects and non-linear association between temperature and mortality (Hajat et al. 2005; Baccini et al. 2008; Rocklov and Forsberg 2008; Gasparrini and Armstrong 2010).

Many studies about temperature-related death showed that the longer lag times are common at cold weather, and shorter lag times are often at hot weather (Armstrong 2006; Anderson and Bell 2009; Martin et al. 2012). As a result, the deaths from high temperature are likely to happen quickly while deaths from low temperature can occur several days after the cold weather. The longer lag times also showed a deficit in mortality if there is mortality displacement associated with the heat stress effects (Kovats and Hajat 2008).

6) Mortality displacement

Possible mortality displacement forward into the hot period or short-term harvesting of death is a key issue when assessing impacts of heat stress on mortality in the time-series studies and particularly the studies of the number of deaths in extreme events such as heat waves (Hajat et al. 2005; Gasparrini and Armstrong 2010; Hajat et al. 2010). It is very important for policy makers to use the evidence-based information of heat stress effects on deaths taking into account the mortality displacement issues (Hajat et al. 2010).

During heat waves, mortality displacement refers to the extreme temperature events that induce a short-term forward shift in the observed mortality distribution among the selected population, or in some locations. The deaths increase during the extreme temperature and then decrease in a few days or weeks later regardless of high heat exposure (Kinney et al. 2008). Here, the mortality displacement affects people who are very near death and have been brought forward by the heat stress effects within a short period of time such as elderly people or those who have chronic diseases (Basu 2009; Hajat et al. 2010). Therefore, the investigation of the heat wave effects on mortality in the time-series analyses should involve the harvesting effects that reduce the overall long-term impacts of heat stress, and should take into account the mortality displacement issue in order to produce accurate estimates (Gasparrini and Armstrong 2010).

2.5 Impacts of future climate change on heat stress-related health outcomes

The global average temperature is expected to continue to increase, which leads to a higher heat stress exposure in the population. The Fourth Assessment Report of the Intergovernmental Panel on Climate Change (IPCC) confirmed that an increase in the global average temperature is very likely to be due to an increase in anthropogenic greenhouse gas concentrations (IPCC 2007). Moreover, the rising global mean temperature will change the climate patterns and temperature variability around the world (IPCC 2007).

The global average temperatures were observed in the past from 1906 to 2005 and showed that many parts of the world have become warmer (IPCC 2007). Overall, the average temperature increased by 0.74°C during the last century (IPCC 2007). The annual global average temperature from 1850 to 1915 was relatively in line with its natural variation. It increased by 0.35°C from the 1910s to the 1940s, and then increased faster by 0.55°C from the 1970s to 2006 with the 11 hottest years during the 1995-2006 period (IPCC 2007).

In addition, the climate warming projected will lead to more hot days and warm nights. The temperature is increasing so that by the end of this century, the global mean temperature could rise in the range of 0.6 to 2.5°C by 2050, and 1.8 to 4.0°C by 2100 (IPCC 2007). In particular for tropical areas, the mean temperature will increase in the range of 1 to 2°C by 2050 and 2 to 4°C by 2090 (IPCC 2007). These changes will expand the heat stress hazards that threaten population health in tropical countries where the health impacts may be exacerbated by high humidity.

The Fourth Assessment Report of the IPCC (2007) indicated that the recent increase in the mean temperature will increase in the mean and tail behaviour of climate event (Figure 2.1). Small increases in the average temperature can make huge changes by reducing in areas of extremely low temperature and increasing in areas with extremely high temperature (IPCC 2001). The hot weather events will increase in duration, frequency and intensity during summer in the future (IPCC 2007).

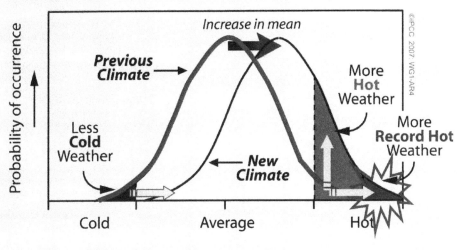

Modified from (IPCC 2007)

Figure 2.1 IPCC schematic depiction of climate change with a shift towards higher temperature

Accordingly, the global population will be exposed to higher levels of heat stress than before and this is likely to have adverse health impacts from climate change (Confalonieri et al. 2007). Substantial health impacts can be a sudden and unpredictable increase in heat-related illness and deaths (Kalkstein 1993; Basu and Samet 2002b; Koppe et al. 2004; Confalonieri et al. 2007; Hajat et al. 2010).

Awareness and public concern about climate change and human health impacts are continuously increasing. The evidence from climate and health relationships confirms that climate change can lead to abrupt or irreversible health outcomes (Confalonieri et al. 2007). However, for the association between climate and health, attributing causality is still unclear. Therefore, there is a need for understanding the potential causes and effects of climate change (Patz et al. 2008). According to McMichael and Githeko (2001), the impacts of climate change on human health can occur via direct and indirect pathways (Figure 2.2).

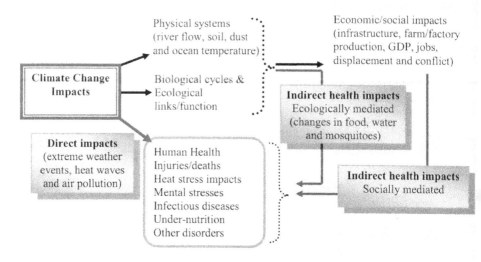

Modified from (McMichael and Githeko 2001)

Figure 2.2 Climate change and human health impact pathways

The indirect health impacts of climate change are complex as they involve ecologically and socially mediated pathways (McMichael and Githeko 2001). The indirect health impacts of climate change are difficult to specify and to investigate because many factors are connected to health in different ways. For example, climate change affects food yields, which has potential effects on malnutrition. Climate change increase extreme weather events such as prolonged droughts, which can impact mental health. Also, climate change is likely to increase abundance of mosquitoes and lead to higher transmission of infectious diseases (Bambrick et al. 2008).

The direct health impacts of climate change are easier to study compared to the indirect health impacts. The studies of health impact assessment from climate change mostly estimate the changes in mortality as a result of increasing temperature in the future (Kalkstein and Greene 1997; Dessai 2003; Gosling et al. 2009a). Those studies quantified the association between the historical temperature variability and mortality over a long period of time. They provide the evidence of an existing heat-related death relationship and then estimate the projected temperature related mortality under climate change scenarios (Gosling et al. 2009b).

Kalkstein and Greene (1997) applied climate change scenarios to estimate the excess mortality in the 44 cities of United States for the year 2020 and 2050. They concluded that the excess mortality will increase attributable to the increased temperature in summer. The total excess mortality of 44 cities will be 1,900-4,000 deaths in 2020, and 3,200-4,700 deaths in 2050 assuming that the population changes in acclimatisation to the increased temperature (Kalkstein and Greene 1997).

In temperate and subtropical countries (such as the United States, the United Kingdom, Australia), the mortality rates are higher in winter than in summer (Kilbourne 2002). An increasing temperature in winter from climate change in such countries would lead to a consistent reduction in cold-related death (Donaldson et al. 2003). For example, a study by Guest et al. (1999) reported that heat-related death would increase among five capital cities in Australia in 2030. However, the climate change will offset a reduction in cold-related mortality and result in an overall reduction of daily heat-related deaths in 2030 by 10% (Guest et al. 1999).

According to the evidence available from previous studies, the predictions of heat stress effects from climate change scenarios are complex and have many uncertainties (McMichael and Githeko 2001; Kinney et al. 2008). Heat-related deaths in summer may be higher than cold-related deaths in winter and would vary among geographic locations and different populations (Kinney et al. 2008). A study based on data from European cities suggests that the association between temperature and mortality are different by latitude (Curriero et al. 2002). Some regions with hotter summers do not have significantly different annual heat-related deaths compared to cold regions.

At this point, the results from previous studies pose a question whether the increasing heat stress from climate change in the future will cause more deaths in summer or reduce more deaths in winter. They also suggested that additional research is needed to understand how heat-related death changes overtime under different plausible scenarios of socio-economic, population demographic, policy interventions, mitigation and adaptation activities and uncertainties from climate model projections (IPCC 2007; Kinney et al. 2008).

This is especially important in tropical developing countries where heat stress has already been a problem. A large number of populations in urban areas are likely to experience health effects from heat stress; this will become more severe from the combined effects of heat stress with urban heat island and air pollution. Therefore, the populations in developing countries will face the higher risks of heat stress effects in the future because climate change will increase the frequency, intensity and duration of heat stress, which will pose serious public health problems.

2.6 Heat stress and climate change in Thailand

The average temperature in Thailand has already increased by around 1°C since 1951 (Thai Meteorological Department 2007). The number of hot days and warm nights has also increased in Thailand (Limsakul and Goes 2008). Thailand is a tropical developing country located in Southeast Asia between latitudes 5° 37'N to 20° 27'N and longitudes 97° 22'E to 105° 37'E (Meteorological Development Bureau 2012). The total area of Thailand is about 514,000 square kilometres with 2,165 kilometres of coastline (National Statistical Office 2011).

The climate characteristics vary among regions of Thailand. The North of Thailand is a mountain area where the hot and cold seasons are very different while the hot and cold seasons in the equatorial South are very similar due to rainfall all year round. Therefore, populations living in different regions are susceptible to different weather variation or different magnitudes of heat stress effects.

2.6.1 Temperature in Thailand

Temperature in Thailand has been increasing from the last 50 years. During 1951 to 2003, the annual average maximum temperature in Thailand increased by 0.56°C and the annual average minimum temperature increased even more by 1.44°C (Limsakul and Goes 2008). Furthermore, the Meteorological Department of Thailand found that the annual average mean, maximum and minimum temperatures had been increasing during 1951 and 2003 (Figure 2.3).

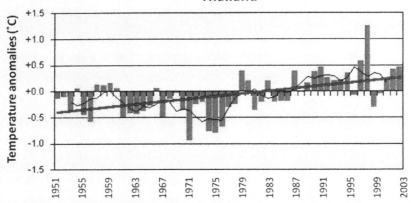

Note: 1) Weather data from 45 weather stations
2) Compared with baseline data from 1971 to 2000

Modified from (Thai Meteorological Department 2007)

Figure 2.3 The annual average maximum temperature in Thailand from 1951 to 2003

In those 50 years, there was an increase in the annual average maximum temperature at around 0.8°C, the annual average minimum temperature at around 1.2°C, and the annual mean temperature by about 1°C (Thai Meteorological Department 2007). These findings from Thai Meteorological Department of the rising temperature are similar to the study reported by Limsakul and Goes (2008).

According to the Bangkok Assessment Report on Climate Change (Sintunawa et al. 2009), the annual average maximum temperature in Thailand was 35°C and there were 121 days when the annual average maximum temperature was over 35°C during 1967 and 2007. Thailand already has a warming temperature and high humidity. The increasing heat stress in the future is anticipated due to the climate change in Thailand (Atsamon et al. 2007).

2.6.2 Climate change situation in Thailand

Meteorological forecasts on the future air temperature in Thailand show that the maximum temperature will increase in many parts across the country. The Southeast Asia START Regional Center (2009) investigated the future climate in Thailand using the PRECIS (Providing Regional Climates for Impact Studies) model and the global dataset of ECHAM4, the model simulation of present-day climate, to project the climate change scenarios between the 2010s and 2090s (SEA START RC 2009). They demonstrated that the increased maximum temperature will widely extend across the country (Figure 2.4).

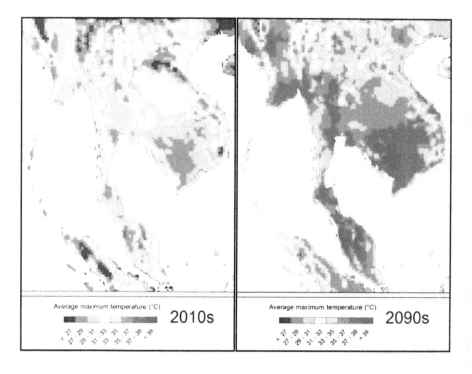

Source (SEA START RC 2009)

Figure 2.4 Average daily maximum temperatures (°C) in Thailand in the 2010s and 2090s

The average daily maximum temperature in the 2010s to 2090s will increase from 34-36°C to 38-40°C (SEA START RC 2009). Moreover, there has been the prediction on the substantial increase in number of days with average maximum temperature exceeding 35°C. The number of hot days is around 150-240 days per year in the 2010s and is expected to increase by 60-90 days in the 2090s (Chidthai-song 2010).

2.7 Awareness about heat stress, climate change and health in Thailand

Recently, climate change in Thailand has received a lot of attention (Marks 2011). The impacts of climate change on Thailand have become increasingly visible as Thais experience increasingly hotter weather (Thai Meteorological Department 2007). This section summarises the national policy responses, some organisations or institutions that deal with climate change in Thailand.

Thailand signed the United Nations Framework Convention on Climate Change (UNFCC) on 28 December 1994 (Office of Natural Resources and Environmental Policy and Planning 2009). Since then several agencies have participated in the climate change issue; especially the government sectors have a vital role to increase public awareness on climate change.

The Ministry of Natural Resources and Environment (MNRE) established the National Committee on Climate Change Policy in August 2006 which replaced the previous Sub-Committee level that was established in 1993 (Office of Natural Resources and Environmental Policy and Planning 2009). Also, there is a new divisional-level office, the Climate Change Coordination Office, established under the Office of Natural Resources and Environmental Policy and Planning (ONEP) to serve as a secretariat of the National Committee on Climate Change Policy, as well as to coordinate the implementing agencies working on the projects related to climate change impact, vulnerability and adaptation (SEA START RC 2009).

In February 2007, the Thai Meteorological Department (TMD) integrated the Climate group and the Climate Academic group at the TMD into the National Climate Center of Thailand (NCCT). The NCCT is a research centre monitoring and preparing the climate early warning system and provides climate information and climate prediction for local and international sectors (Office of Natural Resources and Environmental Policy and Planning 2009).

The Southeast Asia START Regional Center is a research institute working on climate change in Thailand (SEA START RC 2009). It is a non-government research network hosted by NCCT and operated by Chulalongkorn University in Bangkok since 1994. Their research efforts are related to climate change in Thailand including: capacity building for climate adaptation, greenhouse gas mitigation, providing research on adaptation and mitigation, raising public awareness and public participation as well as supporting international cooperation on climate change mitigation.

The changing climate and the rise in the global temperature is predicted to increase adverse health outcomes in the future. Some organisations and research institutes are now working on climate change in term of human health impacts. For example, a research team at Faculty of Public Health, Thammasat University in collaboration with the "High Occupational Temperature: Health and Productivity Suppression" (HOTHAPS) international study (Kjellstrom et al. 2009a) is now working on the climate change and occupational heat stress among Thai workers (Sutthanusorn et al. 2012). Also, the Ministry of Public Health (MOPH) has set up the thematic working group to do research and to coordinate the project of health impact assessment from climate change in Thailand (Department of Health 2009).

Regarding the concern among public health professionals on health and climate change in Thailand, most of the operations emphasise on disease incidence, epidemic conditions, protection and prevention. An understanding of the heat stress-related health outcomes in relation to climate change has tended to receive less attention. Heat-related illness is identified and recorded in the tenth revision of the International Classification of Diseases (ICD-10) in category T67 for the effects of heat and light. A heat-related death is classified according to ICD-10 in the category X30 for excessive natural heat exposure and X32 for sunstroke. Table 2.1 summarises the number of heat-related illness recorded with ICD-10 category T67 in Thailand between 2007 and 2009 (Langkulsen 2011).

Table 2.1 Heat-related illness recorded in the ICD-10 category T67 in Thailand during 2007 and 2009

ICD-10 category T67	Morbidity (person)
T67.0 Heat stroke and sunstroke	94
T67.1 Heat syncope	39
T67.2 Heat cramps	15
T67.3 Heat exhaustion, anhydrotic	1
T67.5 Heat exhaustion, unspecified	30
T67.6 Heat fatigue, transient	33
T67.7 Heat edema	1
T67.8 Other specified heat effects	4
T67.9 Unspecified effects of heat and light	8
Total	**225**

Modified from: (Langkulsen 2011)

For heat-related deaths, the Ministry of Public Health reported four deaths from heat stroke in 2008, three deaths in 2009, 15 deaths during summer in 2010, and eight deaths in 2011 (Sirisawang 2011). It should be noted that many deaths from heat stroke were recorded among Thai soldiers who were trained as draftees in military (Sirisawang 2011). The number of fatal heat strokes in the Thai mortality statistic seems to be underreported. This may be due to fatal heat stroke being similar to other causes of death such as cerebral thrombosis (Keatinge et al. 1986). High temperature is common in Thailand, thus the diagnosis of heat-related illness or causes of death from heat stress are overlooked as the primary cause of illness or death. However, it is still unclear why the Thai mortality records have such a small number of heat-related deaths.

There are very few published studies investigating the association between heat stress and health impacts in Thailand. These studies covered only two metropolitan cities - Bangkok and Chiang Mai (McMichael et al. 2008; Pudpong and Hajat 2011). McMichael et al. (2008) and Guo et al. (2012) found that there is a non-linear relationship between daily mean temperature and non-external deaths. Pudpong and Hajat (2011) found that the diabetic and circulatory visits as well as the hospital admission of intestinal infectious diseases were associated with an increase in the daily mean temperature above the threshold of 29°C in Chiang Mai.

As mentioned previously, little is known on the effects of heat stress on mortality in a tropical environment, especially in Asia (Kovats and Akhtar 2008). Furthermore, the interaction of tropical heat, urbanisation and air pollution as health risk factors is complex and little understood. To address this important knowledge gap, the final section of this chapter summarises the research needs for Thailand.

2.8 Conclusions: research needs for Thailand

The evidence of association between heat stress and health impacts emerged from existing studies in non-tropical developed countries. There are only a few studies conducted in tropical developing countries such as Thailand. There is a need for epidemiological evidence of the heat stress-related health outcomes among the working population and also the overall population as well as the future heat-related deaths from climate change in Thailand.

2.8.1 Heat stress and health impacts among working population in Thailand

Health impact assessment from heat stress exposure should identify the specific risk groups who are most often exposed to heat. Thailand is a middle income tropical country with around 65 million people. Following rapid urbanisation, currently around 46% of the Thai population live in urban areas and it is predicted that by 2030 this will be more than 60% (National Statistical Office 2011). Social and economic transitions in Thailand lead to an increase in the size of the working population (Kelly et al. 2010). More than 39 million are people in the workforce of which more than 16 million are agricultural workers (National Statistical Office 2012).

A study of occupational heat stress in Thailand by Langkulsen et al. (2010) reported that heat stress in Thailand is a very serious problem ("extreme caution" or "danger") in a wide variety of work settings. They tested a pottery factory, a power plant, a knife manufacturing site, a construction site, and an agricultural site. This study indicated that Thai workers in the industrial and agricultural workplaces faced the excessive heat conditions in which heat-related illness are likely to happen (Langkulsen et al. 2010). Another study found that salt production workers in Thailand worked under heat stress where the average temperature in the working environment was 33.8±0.95°C and those workers who worked under heat stress were likely to have heat symptoms compared to unexposed group (Jakreng 2010).

Moreover, workers should be concerned in terms of heat stress effects on health and their productivity because they are often exposed to heat, especially outdoor workers in the tropical developing countries (Kjellstrom 2009b; Kjellstrom et al. 2009a; Kjellstrom et al. 2009b). Those workers carry out heavy work in hot and humid conditions in Thailand and may reach physiological limits to carry out their strenuous work. To avoid the acute heat-related illness or heat stroke, workers have to avoid working during the hottest part of the day, which may lead to the reduction of their work productivity. As a result, they are likely to lose income which can increase their mental stress (Kjellstrom et al. 2009b). Moreover, increasing heat stress exposure from rising temperatures with climate change would make this situation worse.

Thus, heat stress is already a problem in Thailand and there is a need to be more concerned for occupational heat stress problem among Thai workers. As there is a large number of working population from industrial development, demanding-labour works are need and ongoing climate change will lead to higher heat exposures in workers and most likely affect poor people in labouring occupations. Therefore, this thesis will address the unanswered issue of heat stress-related health outcomes among Thai workers by exploring the association between occupational heat stress and health impacts among workers in Thailand.

2.8.2 Heat stress and health impacts among overall Thai population

A large number of people in Thailand have already been exposed to heat beyond the acceptable limits. The rapid economic development and growing urbanisation in Thailand can increase the number of population who are vulnerable to the effects of heat stress. However, there are only few studies of heat stress effects on health and well-being in Thailand. Therefore, there is a need to determine heat stress exposure among Thai populations and to investigate the association between heat stress and health outcomes. These results will be beneficial to the public health and related sectors to prepare the implementations to deal with climate change in the future.

According to the literature review on heat-related death, methods for describing and measuring heat stress effects on mortality are still underdeveloped and many uncertainties remain. There are only a few published studies about heat-related deaths in two cities (Chiang Mai and Bangkok) in Thailand (McMichael et al. 2008; Pudpong and Hajat 2011; Guo et al. 2012), and it leaves questions about the heat stress effects on health of the whole population across the country.

Moreover, effects of air pollution on mortality were found in a few epidemiological studies in Thailand, especially in Bangkok (Vajanapoom et al. 2002; Vichit-Vadakan et al. 2008; Vichit-Vadakan et al. 2010; Wong et al. 2010). Wong at el (2010) and Vichit-Vadakan et al. (2010) presented that the increasing concentrations of particulate matter (PM_{10}) are associated with increasing mortality. Both studies suggested that the high daily mean temperature in tropical Bangkok is a contributing factor. However, the modification effect of heat stress and air pollution on mortality is still unclear and needs further investigation. Therefore, in a later chapter, the study on the association between heat stress and mortality in Thailand needs to take into account of the air pollution effects on the heat stress and mortality relationship.

Research on heat-related death with climate change requires not only exposure–response functions of temperature and mortality, also but information on how these associations differ by geographical locations. The relationship between heat stress and death will be explored in order to present evidence of the heat stress effects on mortality in each region and each season, and also to estimate future heat-related deaths from climate change in Thailand.

2.8.3 Future heat-related death from climate change in Thailand

Recently, the epidemiological studies analyse the heat stress and health relationship, and also estimate the heat-related deaths in the future as a result of climate change (Gosling et al. 2009a). However, many studies about heat-related deaths were conducted in developed and non-tropical regions. This leaves unanswered questions about the effect of heat stress on health in tropical developing countries where temperatures and humidity are already high.

Thailand is a tropical developing country with persistently high temperature and high humidity. Climate change in Thailand is anticipated to bring more hot days and warm nights which can cause impacts to overall population in the future. For human health effects from climate change in Thailand, there is still a lack of information on the effects of future climate change on heat stress-related health outcomes. Consequently, there is a need to investigate and to assess the potential impacts of climate change on human health in Thailand. It is important to raise awareness of the population regarding climate change in order to minimise the impacts and to cope with the consequences of climate change. Also, this research will be useful for policy makers and related sectors to prevent adverse heat stress-related health outcomes from future climate change.

CHAPTER 3: HEAT STRESS AND MENTAL HEALTH[1]

Heat stress is a problem in Thailand where there are often high temperatures and high humidity. Over 70% of the Thai population in a large national Thai Cohort Study (TCS) are workers who may be vulnerable to heat stress effect due to frequent exposure to heat from their job. They also carry out heavy labour outdoors or indoors without air conditioning. The TCS project was established in 2005 to study the health-risk transition of a large national cohort of adult Thais and they are available to investigate the association between heat stress and health outcomes in Thailand. There are very few recent studies which have reported on the association of occupational heat stress and mental health or overall health in workers. However, the socioeconomic development and rapid urbanisation in tropical developing countries such as Thailand creates working conditions in which heat stress is likely. Hence, this study aims at identifying the relationship between self-reported heat stress and psychological distress and overall health in Thai workers.

[1] A version of Chapter 3 has been published. Tawatsupa B, Lim LL-Y, Kjellstrom T, Seubsman S, Sleigh A, the Thai Cohort Study team (2010) The association between overall health, psychological distress, and occupational heat stress among a large national cohort of 40,913 Thai workers. *Global Health Action* 3. DOI: 10.3402/gha.v3i0.5034

CO_ACTION

The association between overall health, psychological distress, and occupational heat stress among a large national cohort of 40,913 Thai workers

Benjawan Tawatsupa[1,2*], Lynette L-Y. Lim[2], Tord Kjellstrom[2], Sam-ang Seubsman[3], Adrian Sleigh[2] and the Thai Cohort Study team[3,a]

[1]Health Impact Assessment Division, Department of Health, Ministry of Public Health, Thailand; [2]National Centre for Epidemiology and Population Health, The Australian National University, Canberra, Australia; [3]Thai Health-Risk Transition: a National Cohort Study, Sukhothai Thammathirat Open University, Nonthaburi, Thailand

Background: Occupational heat stress is a well-known problem, particularly in tropical countries, affecting workers, health and well-being. There are very few recent studies that have reported on the effect of heat stress on mental health, or overall health in workers, although socioeconomic development and rapid urbanization in tropical developing countries like Thailand create working conditions in which heat stress is likely.

Objective: This study is aimed at identifying the relationship between self-reported heat stress and psychological distress, and overall health status in Thai workers.

Results: 18% of our large national cohort (>40,000 subjects) often works under heat stress conditions and males are exposed to heat stress more often than females. Furthermore, working under heat stress conditions is associated with both worse overall health and psychological distress (adjusted odds ratios ranging from 1.49 to 1.84).

Conclusions: This association between occupational heat stress and worse health needs more public health attention and further development on occupational health interventions as climate change increases Thailand's temperatures.

Keywords: *occupational heat stress; psychological distress; poor overall health; Thailand*

Received: 29 January 2010; Revised: 1 April 2010; Accepted: 19 April 2010; Published: 13 May 2010

E xposure to extreme heat conditions has been found to be hazardous to health and has been linked in many studies to a range of illnesses and premature death (1–4). Workers frequently exposed to heat in their workplace have been found to suffer heat exhaustion, heat stroke, kidney disease, heart or lung disease, accidents, and injuries (5–8). This is especially true for those people whose occupation involves performing physical labor outdoors, who are exposed to higher-than-normal ambient temperatures combined with the body heat generated by the jobs themselves (7, 9).

Factors such as pre-existing disease, clothing, age, gender, ability for heat acclimatization, level of physical activity, and body size, can influence the health impact of heat stress (6, 10, 11). Moreover, socioeconomic factors such as income and urbanization can compound the adverse health outcomes from heat stress (9). For

[a]*Thailand*: Jaruwan Chokhanapitak, Chaiyun Churewong, Suttanit Hounthasarn, Suwanee Khamman, Daoruang Pandee, Suttinan Pangsap, Tippawan Prapamontol, Janya Puengson, Yodyiam Sangrattanakul, Sam-ang Seubsman, Boonchai Somboonsook, Nintita Sripaiboonkij, Pathumvadee Somsamai, Duangkae Vilainerun, Wanee Wimonwattanaphan. *Australia:* Chris Bain, Emily Banks, Cathy Banwell, Bruce Caldwell, Gordon Carmichael, Tarie Dellora, Jane Dixon, Sharon Friel, David Harley, Matthew Kelly, Tord Kjellstrom, Lynette Lim, Anthony McMichael, Tanya Mark, Adrian Sleigh, Lyndall Strazdins, Vasoontara Yiengprugsawan.

example, poor farmers and laborers are at greatest risk of heat stress due to prolonged heat exposure during hot days, in contrast to urban workers who have middle or high incomes, and are likely to install air conditioning in their dwellings and offices (7). Additionally, infrastructure, buildings, roads, and other major physical structures capture and absorb solar heat radiation in urban areas, causing the temperature to rise faster and to higher levels than in rural areas because of the 'urban heat island effect' (12), thus laborers in urban areas may experience the largest temperature-related health risk.

Kjellstrom et al. (7) have identified the potential occupational health problems that climate change and associated increased heat exposure might cause, especially in low- and middle-income countries in tropical areas. For example, heat stroke has been reported among laborers in gold mines in South Africa, and heat stress has been noticed to lower productivity among female workers in a shoe factory in Vietnam (9). They suggest that more research is needed on links between heat stress and adverse health outcomes in working populations, especially in developing countries.

We have conducted such preliminary research in Thailand, a tropical developing country with a large working population commonly exposed to heat with both high air temperature and humidity, particularly during the hot season. Moreover, the mean temperature in Thailand has already increased 0.74°C in the past 40 years, and it is expected that extreme temperature events will become more prevalent in the future (13). However, heat effects on health have received little attention in Thailand and there are very few studies on occupational heat stress and heat-related illness (6, 14) and no published studies report on the effects of heat stress at work on mental health in the Thai context.

Berry et al. (15) illustrated that the increasing heat exposure on workers in tropical countries as an effect of climate change may indirectly cause psychological distress in workers due to reduced work productivity, lost income, and disrupted daily social activity. Therefore, here we present an analysis of self-reported mental and overall health and their association with heat stress among workers in a large national cohort study underway in Thailand. We also note the influence of age, sex, job type and location, income, education, and other work hazards among a group experiencing socioeconomic development, rapid urbanization, demanding jobs, and long working hours in hot conditions.

Methodology

Data

The data derive from the baseline measurements of a large national Thai Cohort Study (TCS) that began in 2005, researching the health-risk transition in the adult

Thai population. The study began with a 20-page mailout questionnaire covering social demography, work, health and injuries, social networks and well-being, diet and physical activity, and tobacco, alcohol, and transport. There were 87,134 respondents aged 15–87 years enrolled as distance learning students at Sukhothai Thammathirat Open University (STOU). Further details about the questionnaire data collection and the attributes of respondents are given in Sleigh et al. (16).

Measurements

The information on individual experiences of heat stress was derived from the question: 'During the last 12 months, how often have you experienced at work high temperatures which make you uncomfortable?', which 76,113 respondents answered on a four-point scale ('often,' 'sometimes,' 'rarely,' and 'never'). For analysis, self-reported occupational heat stress was dichotomized into often or not often.

Outcomes assessed were self-reported poor overall health and psychological distress. Poor overall health is based on the first question of the Medical Outcomes short form instrument (SF8) – 'overall how would you rate your health during the past four weeks (excellent, very good, good, fair, poor, or very poor).' For analysis, we combined the last two categories as 'poor overall health' and the first four categories as 'not poor overall health.' Psychological distress is based on the three anxiety-oriented questions of the standard Kessler 6 psychological distress questions: 'in the past 4 weeks, about how often did you feel ...(nervous, restless or fidgety, or everything was an effort)' with answers on a five-point scale (1 = all of the time, 2 = most of the time, 3 = some of the time, 4 = a little of the time, 5 = none of the time). For our analysis, if the average response for the three questions was less than or equal to 2, the respondent was classified as psychologically distressed.

The population hierarchy for participant analysis is shown in Fig. 1. Overall, most of those excluded did not answer the questions regarding work or were not working in paid employment for at least 40 hours per week. All respondents reported age, sex, education, income, location of job, job type, and five other hazards at work (beside high temperature); data on these variables were collected because they could confound or modify our estimates of the association between overall health, psychological distress, and occupational heat stress.

For analysis, age in years was divided into three categories (15–29, 30–44, >45), highest education was divided into three categories (high school, diploma, or university), monthly income (in Thai Baht) was divided into four categories ('up to 7,000,' '7,001–10,000,' '10,001–20,000,' and '20,001 and more'), and job location was divided into three categories (Bangkok, urban-outside Bangkok, and rural). Some analyses were restricted

Citation: Global Health Action 2010, 3: 5034 - DOI: 10.3402/gha.v3i0.5034

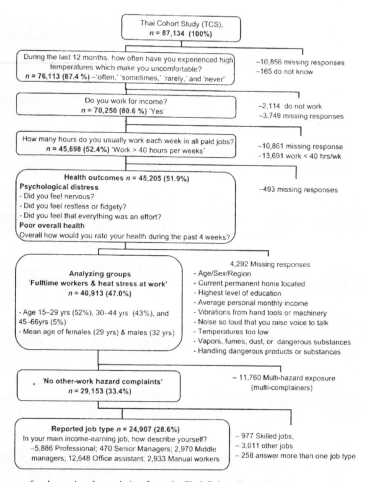

Fig. 1. Selection process for the analyzed population from the Thai Cohort Study data.

to the population providing information on job type categorized as office job or physical job (those reporting as 'skilled workers' were excluded because we could not categorize them further). Complaints about five other hazards at work (vibrations from tools or machines, loud noise, uncomfortably low temperatures, dangerous fumes (vapors, chemicals, infectious agents), and touching dangerous substances) were each also categorized as often/not often and the 'often' results combined into three levels (0 other complaints, 1–2 other complaints, 3–5 other complaints).

Data analysis
Data were digitized using Thai Scandevet software and further processed using SPSS and Stata statistical packages. The initial analysis group included 40,913 fulltime workers for overall heat stress analyses. Final

heat stress analyses were restricted to the 24,907 workers whose job type was known (allowing assessment of this variable) and who did not make non-thermal work hazard complaints (preventing any influence on the results of adverse effects of 'multiple hazard complainers').

Summary statistics (means and proportions by variable category and sex) were prepared for heat stress, age, education, income, job, and work hazard complaints. All explanatory variables (i.e. sex, age, job location, job type, education, income, other work hazards) were assessed as potential confounders of our estimates of heat stress associations on health outcomes by investigating their association with the exposure of interest (heat stress) or the outcomes (overall health or psychological distress). Both outcomes were assessed graphically for association with heat stress and these analyses were broken down by age group (15–29, 30–44, >45 years) and sex.

The association between heat stress and overall health or psychological distress was assessed by odds ratios (ORs) and 95% confidence intervals. Using multivariable logistic regression, these heat stress ORs were adjusted for the influence of all confounding variables (sex, age, job type, job location, education, income, and complaints of other work hazards). These variables were also evaluated as potential modifiers of heat stress associations by stratified analyses that estimated the ORs separately for each category (i.e. by sex, age group, education group, income group, complaint group, job location, job type and by the joint effect of job type and location). Each stratified OR was adjusted for the confounding influence of other explanatory variables (e.g. sex, age group, etc.).

Finally, using stepwise logistic regression to include only significant confounders and heat stress interaction terms, models were prepared to show the fully adjusted heat stress association on overall health and on psychological distress. The final model for the 40,913 fulltime workers for overall health included heat stress, sex, age, education, other complaints, job location, and two interaction terms (education × heat, and other complaints × heat). The final model for psychological distress included heat stress, sex, age, education, income, other complaints, job location, and an interaction term for other complaints × heat. When job type was offered for the stepwise models and these workers were potentially exposed to heat stress only (restricted data set, $n = 24,907$), the final model for both poor health and psychological distress included heat stress, sex, age, and job location. There were no significant interaction terms in these final models linking heat stress to either health outcome.

Ethical issues
Ethical approval was obtained from STOU Research Committee and the Australian National University Human Research Ethics Committee (ANU HREC). Informed written consent was obtained from all participants.

Results

Characteristics of the cohort
Tables 1 and 2, and Fig. 1 present the main characteristics of all 40,913 Thai cohort members who were fulltime workers. Overall, 56% were female. More than half the cohort was young, aged between 15 and 29 years (52%). Nearly 20% of workplaces were located in Bangkok, 41% were in other urban areas (outside Bangkok), and 39% were in rural areas, 19% of classifiable jobs were physical and 81% were based in an office. Compared with males, females were younger and worked in Bangkok (22 vs 17%).

On average, women had moderately higher educational achievements whereas men had substantially higher personal incomes. Overall, 5% of fulltime workers reported often experiencing three to five other hazards beside high temperature at work, more for males (6%) than females (3%). Over 18% ($n = 7,476$) of the analyzed group reported they often experienced uncomfortably high temperatures at work (Table 2). This problem was worse for males (23%) than females (15%); also females more frequently than males reported never experiencing heat stress at work (27 vs 17%).

Associations of cohort attributes with heat stress, overall health, and psychological distress
Heat stress exposure together with health and psychological distress outcomes are summarized in Table 3. Here we explore the associations of heat stress exposures and health outcomes with potential confounders of the heat stress effects. The prevalence of heat stress ('often' experiencing high temperatures at work ($n = 40,913$)) varied considerably among subgroups and was notably high for those with other complaints regarding hazards at work. Nearly 5% of workers reported poor overall health and this figure rose to 9% for those reporting often being troubled by three to five other work hazards. Psychological distress was more common; overall, it affected 8% of workers and was reported by 20% of those with three to five other work hazards.

In almost all instances the potential confounders shown in Table 3 (sex, age group, education, income, job type, job location, and other work hazard complaints) were significantly associated with both the exposure of interest (heat stress) and the two outcomes (overall health and psychological distress). Accordingly, our analyses of heat stress effects were adjusted for these confounding variables, or restricted to exclude all those respondents who had multiple work hazard complaints.

Effect of heat stress on overall health and psychological distress
Figs. 2 and 3 reveal the positive association between heat stress and poor health or psychological distress stratified by age group and sex. This analysis was restricted to the 24,907 workers who did not complain of multiple work hazards and whose job type was known. The association between overall health, psychological distress, and occupational heat stress are substantial and revealed no consistent pattern with age. Generally, the adverse effects of heat stress on poor health were worse for females; the opposite association was noted for heat stress and psychological distress, which was especially bad for males aged between 15 and 29 years.

Citation: Global Health Action 2010, **3**: 5034 - DOI: 10.3402/gha.v3i0.5034

Table 1. Socioeconomic and other attributes in a cohort of 40,913 fulltime workers in Thailand

Attributes	Male n	Male %	Female n	Female %	Total n	Total %
Total	18,148	44.7	22,765	55.6	40,913	100.0
Job location						
Bangkok	3,117	17.2	4,961	21.8	8,078	19.7
Urban	7,682	42.3	8,955	39.3	16,637	40.7
Rural	7,349	40.5	8,849	38.9	16,198	39.6
Job type[a]						
Office	11,708	81.0	17,042	85.2	28,750	83.4
Physical	2,741	19.0	2,970	14.8	5,711	16.6
Education						
University	5,271	29.0	6,925	30.4	12,196	29.8
Diploma	4,900	27.0	8,208	36.1	13,108	32.0
High school	7,977	44.0	7,632	33.5	15,609	38.2
Personal income (Baht/month)						
20,001+	2,554	14.1	1,930	8.5	4,484	11.0
10,001–20,000	6,353	35.0	5,862	25.7	12,215	29.9
7,001–10,000	5,121	28.2	6,626	29.1	11,747	28.7
<7,000	4,120	22.7	8,347	36.7	12,467	30.5
Other work hazard complaints						
No other complaints	12,669	69.8	16,484	72.4	29,153	71.3
Scored 1–2 items with 'often'	4,436	24.4	5,501	24.2	9,937	24.3
Scored 3–5 items with 'often'	1,043	5.8	780	3.4	1,823	4.5
Overall health						
No poor overall health	17,484	96.3	21,503	94.5	38,987	95.3
Poor overall health	664	3.8	1,262	5.6	1,926	4.7
Psychological distress						
Not psychologically distressed	16,807	92.6	20,714	90.99	37,521	91.71
Psychologically distressed	1,341	7.4	2,051	9.0	3,392	8.3

[a]Job type is available for analysis with 24,907 respondents (see Section 'Methods').

Modifications of the heat stress effects are summarized in Table 4. For both outcomes, the heat stress effects are increased for workers aged more than 45 years and for the better educated, and for work located in rural areas, but none of these interactions are strong. Perhaps the most notable interaction is the attenuation of heat stress associations among those with multiple work hazard complaints; for example, the association of heat stress

Table 2. Reported heat stress at work in a cohort of 40,913 fulltime workers in Thailand

Sex	Often n	Often %	Sometimes n	Sometimes %	Rarely n	Rarely %	Never n	Never %	Total n	Total %
Males	4,081	22.5	6,187	34.1	4,743	26.1	3,137	17.3	18,148	44.4
Females	3,395	14.9	6,479	28.5	6,789	29.8	6,102	26.8	22,765	55.6
Total	7,476	18.2	12,666	30.9	11,532	28.3	9,239	22.6	40,913	100

Table 3. Heat stress, poor overall health, and psychological distress by potential confounding factors in a cohort of 40,913 fulltime workers

	Heat stress			Poor overall health			Psychological distress		
	%	OR[a]	95% CI	%	OR[a]	95% CI	%	OR[a]	95% CI
Total	18.3			4.7			8.3		
Sex									
Males	22.5	1		3.8	1		7.4	1	
Females	14.9	0.60**	0.57–0.63	5.6	1.55**	1.40–1.70	9.0	1.24**	1.16–1.35
Age group (%)									
15–29	18.2	1		5.1	1		9.9	1	
30–44	18.6	1.02	0.97–1.07	4.5	0.87*	0.79–0.95	6.7	0.65**	0.60–0.70
>45	16.4	0.88*	0.78–0.99	3.9	0.71*	0.56–0.90	4.3	0.41**	0.33–0.52
Job location									
Bangkok	14.0	1		5.8	1		9.5	1	
Urban	18.6	1.39**	1.30–1.50	4.8	0.81*	0.72–0.92	8.3	0.86*	0.78–0.95
Rural	20.1	1.54**	1.43–1.66	4.1	0.70**	0.62–0.79	7.7	0.80**	0.72–0.88
Job type[b]									
Office	10.6	1		3.9	1		6.6	1	
Physical	14.3	1.40**	1.26–1.57	3.8	0.99	0.81–1.21	6.4	0.97	0.83–1.14
Education									
University	15.3	1		4.9	1		7.8	1	
Diploma	17.1	1.14**	1.06–1.22	4.7	0.99	0.88–1.11	8.9	1.16*	1.06–1.28
High school	21.6	1.52**	1.43–1.62	4.8	0.96	0.86–1.09	8.2	1.05	0.97–1.62
Personal income (Baht/month)									
20,001 +	12.6	1		4.4	1		5.8	1	
10,001–20,000	18.1	1.54**	1.39–1.70	4.5	0.99	0.83–1.17	7.1	1.26*	1.09–1.47
7,001–10,000	18.9	1.62**	1.46–1.78	5.0	1.16	0.98–1.37	8.8	1.56**	1.36–1.81
<7,000	19.9	1.73**	1.57–1.91	5.1	1.17	0.98–1.38	9.9	1.77**	1.55–2.06
Other work hazard complaints									
No other complaints	11.4	1		3.9	1		6.3	1	
Scored 1–2 items with 'often'	30.9	3.47**	3.32–3.67	6.7	1.75**	1.59–1.92	12.1	2.05**	1.91–2.24
Scored 3–5 items with 'often'	59.4	11.34**	10.26–12.54	8.9	2.48**	2.09–2.94	19.5	3.60**	3.13–4.06

[a]Associations with heat stress, poor overall health, and psychological distress each expressed as crude odds ratios (ORs).
[b]Job type analysis is restricted to 24,907 respondents (see Section 'Methods').
*$P < 0.05$; **$P < 0.001$.

and overall health (OR = 1.75) compares to an OR of 1.22 for those with three to five complaints.

Table 5 shows crude and adjusted OR estimates for associations between heat stress and poor health and psychological distress outcomes. The adjusted ORs derive from models that include age, sex, income, education, job location, and other work hazard complaints. Cohort members who experienced heat stress at work had higher odds of poor overall health (crude OR = 1.67, P-value <0.001; adjusted OR = 1.49, P-value <0.001). They also had higher odds of psychological distress (crude OR = 2.22, P <0.001; adjusted OR = 1.84,

P-value <0.001). For workers who did not complain of other work hazards and for whom job type was reported (n = 24,907), the adjusted heat stress models ORs for poor health (1.80) and psychological distress (2.19) differ little from previous estimates.

The final logistic regression models included all significant confounders and all significant interactors (see Section 'Methods' and footnote of Table 5). The final ORs linking heat stress to poor overall health were 1.55 (n = 40,913) and 1.81 (when restricted to those reporting job type and no other work hazard complaints, n = 24,907). For psychological distress, the corresponding

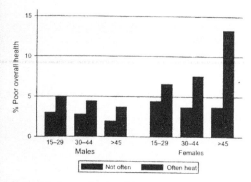

Fig. 2. Prevalence of reported 'poor overall health' by age group, sex, and reported occupational heat stress in 24,907 Thai workers.

final adjusted ORs were similar for the two analytical groups (2.21 for $n = 40,913$ and 2.17 for $n = 24,907$). Accordingly, these final models show considerable and consistent strength of association between heat stress and health outcomes, and the confidence limits and p-values show results unlikely to be due to chance.

Discussion

Statement of principal findings
These findings add to the limited literature on the association between overall health, psychological distress, and occupational heat stress of Thai workers (17). We found heat stress exposure reported by nearly 20% of our large national cohort, more frequently among laborers and male workers, those with low incomes and low education, and declining with age possibly due to an age-related shift away from physical work. Occupational heat stress was reported less frequently in Bangkok, probably reflecting air conditioning in Thai cities, especially in Bangkok (9).

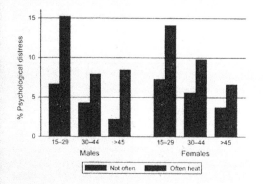

Fig. 3. Prevalence of reported 'psychological distress' by age group, sex, and reported occupational heat stress in 24,907 Thai workers.

The proportion of male workers who reported poor health and psychological distress declined with age. This was especially noteworthy for psychological distress, possibly reflecting longer work experience and the ability to control emotions among older men. For women, the trend of less psychological distress with advancing age was similar. However, heat-stressed females did show a trend of worsening overall health with increasing age, which may reflect aging as well as more responsibilities and daily stress from the mix of professional work and homemaking once a family has formed. This finding is similar to Lennon (1995), who found that women have substantially higher psychological distress than men (18). However, in our study, men aged between 15 and 29 years reported the highest prevalence of distress (Fig. 3), which may be linked to the high rates of suicide and distress in young men in Thailand (19).

Our principal finding is that heat stress was strongly and significantly associated with both poor overall health and psychological distress, with adjusted ORs ranging from 1.49 to 1.84. These epidemiological associations remained substantial and highly significant statistically when extensively adjusted for confounding (by age, sex, income, education, and job location) and when restricted to those who did not have other (non-thermal) work hazard complaints (i.e. non-complainers). The strength of association between overall health, psychological distress, and occupational heat stress interacts weakly with an array of other sociodemographic variables. However, none of the interactions significantly modified the heat stress associations.

Strengths and weaknesses of the study
Access to a large national cohort of 40,913 Thai workers is the main advantage of this study. It represents working-age Thais reasonably well for geographic location, age, sex, and socioeconomic status (16). Cohort members are better educated than average Thais of the same age and sex, but this difference enabled us to gather complex heat exposure and health outcomes on large numbers by questionnaire. This is the first time such a study has been attempted. The cohort shows a wide range of values for the variables of interest, allowing us to investigate the relationship between heat stress at work and health outcomes.

Furthermore, we can be reassured of our results by the restricted analyses of 24,907 workers with all the multi-complainers excluded and job types known. The results are similar to the overall analysis of 40,913 cohort members that was adjusted for confounding and interaction. However, this study could not directly establish that these overall health problems and psychological distress arose as a result of heat stress. There are some difficulties in interpreting these data on exposure patterns and associated health outcomes given that we cannot be

Table 4. Stratified odds ratios revealing interaction of demographic and work-related variables with the association between overall health, psychological distress, and occupational heat stress ($n = 40,913$)

Variables	Heat stress (n)[a]	Poor overall health		Psychological distress	
		OR[b]	95% CI	OR[b]	95% CI
Sex					
Males	4,081	1.40**	1.17–1.69	1.95**	1.72–2.22
Females	3,395	1.55**	1.35–1.79	1.78**	1.59–1.99
Age group					
15–29	3,906	1.38**	1.18–1.60	1.80**	1.62–2.01
30–44	3,234	1.57**	1.31–1.87	1.86**	1.62–2.14
>45	336	1.83*	1.05–3.18	2.35*	1.42–3.88
Education					
University	1,867	1.94**	1.58–2.37	2.04**	1.73–2.40
Diploma	2,240	1.26*	1.02–1.55	1.85**	1.60–2.15
High school	3,369	1.38*	1.15–1.66	1.70**	1.48–1.94
Income					
20,001+	563	1.76*	1.20–2.57	1.99**	1.42–2.77
10,001–20,000	2,214	1.55**	1.24–1.92	1.74**	1.47–2.06
7,001–10,000	2,215	1.39*	1.13–1.72	1.71**	1.47–2.00
<7,000	2,484	1.46**	1.20–1.77	1.99**	1.73–2.28
Complaint effect					
No other complaints	3,324	1.75**	1.49–2.06	2.21**	1.96–2.49
Scored 1–2 items with 'often'	3,070	1.33*	1.12–1.58	1.54**	1.36–1.75
Scored 3–5 items with 'often'	1,082	1.22*	0.87–1.71	1.80**	1.39–2.32
Job location					
Bangkok	1,133	1.36*	1.06–1.76	1.88**	1.55–2.29
Urban	3,089	1.49**	1.25–1.77	1.75**	1.54–2.00
Rural	3,254	1.53**	1.27–1.84	1.90**	1.66–2.18
Job type[c]					
Physical	420	1.91*	1.21–3.00	1.87*	1.30–2.68
Office	2,338	1.79**	1.48–2.15	2.24**	1.94–2.58
Job location/type[c]					
Bangkok/office	251	2.41**	1.52–3.80	2.62**	1.84–3.74
Bangkok/physical	58	0.91	0.25–3.18	1.10	0.36–3.38
Urban/office	945	1.84**	1.37–2.45	2.04**	1.62–2.56
Urban/physical	150	2.32*	1.13–4.75	1.41	0.75–2.65
Rural/office	1,142	1.55*	1.15–2.07	2.35**	1.90–2.90
Rural/physical	212	2.15*	1.08–4.28	2.49**	1.50–4.11

[a]Number of respondents who reported heat stress at work (see Section 'Methods').
[b]Odds ratios show within-strata estimates for heat stress associations adjusted for all other explanatory variables.
[c]Job type analysis restricted to 24,907 respondents (see 'Methods').
*$P < 0.05$; **$P < 0.001$.

sure that heat stress preceded adverse outcomes. Moreover, the source or nature of the heat stress or the work situations was not categorized in this study. Indeed, we were not able to make a direct measurement of work environments or health outcomes, hence we must classify this study as preliminary in nature. Therefore, there is need for more detailed direct observations in informative

work settings to validate our findings and explore the underlying mechanisms.

We were able to find only one other study (an unpublished thesis) of thermal environment and mental health in Thailand, among a small population of 90 workers in a seafood factory (17). This factory study did not document heat stress (but did measure temperature);

Citation: Global Health Action 2010, 3: 5034 - DOI: 10.3402/gha.v3i0.5034

Table 5. The association between occupational heat stress, overall health, and psychological distress

		Poor overall health		Psychological distress	
	Heat stress	OR	95% CI	OR	95% CI
Heat stress (crude estimate)					
$n = 40{,}913$	Not often	1		1	
	Often	1.67**	1.50–1.85	2.22**	2.06–2.40
All variables (adjusted)[a]					
$n = 40{,}913$	Not often	1		1	
	Often	1.49**	1.32–1.66	1.84**	1.69–2.00
All variables (adjusted)[a]					
Restricted $n = 24{,}907$	Not often	1		1	
	Often	1.80**	1.51–2.14	2.19**	1.92–2.50
Final models					
Final model includes interact terms[b]					
$n = 40{,}913$	Not often	1		1	
	Often	1.55**	1.87–3.38	2.21**	1.89–2.37
Final model[c]					
Restricted $n = 24{,}907$	Not often	1		1	
	Often	1.81**	1.52–2.15	2.17**	1.90–2.48

*$P < 0.05$; **$P < 0.001$.
[a]Adjusted ORs derived from heat stress models that included sex, age, income, education, job location, and complaints ($n = 40{,}913$) plus job type ($n = 24{,}907$).
[b]Final model for estimating the association between heat stress and poor overall health includes all statistically significant confounders (sex, age, education, complaints, job location), and the two significant interaction terms (education × heat and complaints × heat). Final model for estimating the association between heat stress and psychological distress includes all statistically significant confounders (sex, age, education, income, complaints, job location) and the one significant interaction term (complaints × heat).
[c]Final model in restricted group ($n = 24{,}907$) for association between heat stress and both poor overall health and psychological distress includes all statistically significant confounders (sex, age, and job location).

nor did it find evidence of widespread psychological distress. Although, there are reports on occupational heat exposure and comfort of workers, they do not usually mention psychological distress or mental health problems as a variable (11, 14). Therefore, our study is one of the first to provide evidence on an association between heat stress and psychological distress of workers.

Significance of this study
This is the first large-scale study of occupational heat stress and adverse health outcomes in Thailand. The findings of widespread heat stress and associated ill-health are disturbing. This is particularly important at present because we can expect that the existing problem will worsen if global warming continues and workplaces become even more thermally stressful. Given the con-strained resources in middle-income Thailand, and the possibility that psychologically stressful work is becom-ing more widespread, our results on psychological distress are of particular concern. If workers exposed to excessive heat cannot cool down, they can experience severe psychological distress caused by heat-related exhaustion or develop long-term conditions such as chronic depression or chronic anxiety disorders (11, 20). Furthermore, Ramsey (21) reported that heat stress diminished mental ability and increased injury risks, and others have noted increased suicide risk (15, 22, 23).

Future research
Occupational heat stress requires more public health attention. Further studies are needed to accurately characterize workplace humidity, air movement, radiant temperature, health outcomes, and work performance in various settings in Thailand, especially as the workforce structure changes with economic development (24, 25).

Acknowledgements

We thank the staff at Sukhothai Thammathirat Open University (STOU) who assisted with student contact and the STOU students who are participating in the cohort study. We also thank Dr Bandit

Thinkamrop and his team from Khon Kaen University for guiding us successfully through the complex data processing.

Conflict of interest and funding

This study was supported by the International Collaborative Research Grants Scheme with joint grants from the Wellcome Trust UK (GR0587MA) and the Australian NHMRC (268055).

References

1. Kovats S, Akhtar R. Climate, climate change and human health in Asian cities. Environ Urban 2008; 20: 165–75.
2. Kovats R, Campbell-Lendrum D, Matthies F. Climate change and human health: estimating avoidable deaths and disease. Risk Anal 2005; 25: 1409–18.
3. McMichael A, McGeehin, Mirabelli M. The potential impacts of climate variability and change on temperature-related morbidity and mortality in the United States. Environ Health Perspect 2001; 9: 185–9.
4. Martens W. Climate change, thermal stress and mortality changes. Soc Sci Med 1998; 46: 331–44.
5. Centers for Disease Control and Prevention. Fatalities from occupational heat exposure. Morbidity and Mortality Weekly Report 1984. Available from http://www.cdc.gov/mmwr/preview/mmwrhtml/00000376.htm [cited 24 April 2009].
6. Chawsithiwong B. Occupational thermal exposure. Thai J Environ Manage 2008; 4: 1–26.
7. Kjellstrom T, Gabrysch S, Lemke B, Dear K. The "Hothaps" program for assessing climate change impacts on occupational health and productivity: an invitation to carry out field studies. Global Health Action 2009; 2. Available from: http://www.globalhealthaction.net/index.php/gha/article/view/2082/2561 [cited 19 April 2010].
8. Rosenstock L, Cullen M. Textbook of clinical occupational and environmental medicine. New York: W.B. Saunders Company; 1994.
9. Kjellstrom T. Climate change, direct heat exposure, health and well-being in low and middle-income countries. Global Health Action 2009; 2: 1–3.
10. Occupational Safety and Health Administration. Heat Stress OSHA Standard. Available from http://www.osha.gov/SLTC/heatstress/standards.html [cited 25 June 2009].
11. Schneider J. Identification and management of thermal stress and strain. Paper presented at Queensland Mining Industry Health and Safety Conference Proceedings, Central Queensland University, 1999.
12. USEPA. Heat island effect. Available from http://www.epa.gov/heatislands [cited 20 October 2009].
13. Limsakul A, Limjirakan S, Sriburi T. Trends in daily temperature extremes in Thailand. Paper presented at the Second National Conference on Natural Resources and Environment, Bangkok, Thailand, 2009.
14. Taptagaporn S, Vichit-Vadakan N, Langkulsen U. Climate change impacts on occupational health in South-East Asia – a preliminary analysis based on data from Thailand. Bangkok: Faculty of Public Health, Thammasat University; 2009.
15. Berry HL, Bowen K, Kjellström T. Climate change and mental health: a causal pathways framework. Int J Public Health 2010; 55: 123–32.
16. Sleigh A, Seubsman S, Bain C, Thai cohort team. Cohort profile: the Thai cohort of 87,134 open university students. Int J Epidemiol 2008; 37: 266–72.
17. Vivatpong Y. Effects of temperature on worker's health and working behavior in sea-food processing factories. Bangkok: Department of Psychology, Kasetsart University; 1995. (In Thai with English abstract.)
18. Lennon MC. Work conditions as explanations for the relation between socioeconomic status, gender, and psychological disorders. Epidemiol Rev 1995; 17: 120–7.
19. Lotrakul M. Suicide in Thailand during the period 1998–2003. Psychiatry Clin Neurosci 2006; 60: 90–5.
20. Hansen A, Bi P, Nitschke M, Ryan P, Pisaniello D, Tucker G. The effect of heat waves on mental health in a temperate Australian city. Environ Health Perspect 2008; 116: 1369–75.
21. Ramsey JD. Task performance in heat: a review. Ergonomics 1995; 38: 154–65.
22. Anderson C. Heat and violence. Curr Direct Psychol Sci 2001; 10: 33–8.
23. Page LA, Hajat S, Kovats RS. Relationship between daily suicide counts and temperature in England and Wales. Br J Psychiatry 2007; 191: 106–12.
24. Kelly M, Strazdins L, Dellora T, Seubsman S, Sleigh A. Thailand's work and health transition. Int Labour Rev 2010 (in press, accepted October 2009).
25. National Statistical Office. Report of the labour force survey. Whole kingdom quarter 4: October–December 2005. Available from http://web.nso.go.th/eng/stat/lfs_e/lfse-tab1.xls [cited 22 June 2009].

*Benjawan Tawatsupa
National Centre for Epidemiology and Population Health
Building 62, The Australian National University
Canberra, ACT 0200, Australia
Tel: +61 2 6125 5615
Fax: +61 2 6125 0740
Email: benjawan.tawatsupa@anu.edu.au

CHAPTER 4: HEAT STRESS AND INJURY[2]

Global warming will increase heat stress at work. The heat stress impacts may arise from increased mistakes in daily activities and lead to accidental injuries. Few studies have addressed the health consequences of heat stress in tropical low and middle income settings such as Thailand. This chapter reports on the association between heat stress and workplace injury among workers enrolled in the large national Thai Cohort Study in 2005. This study used the TCS data at baseline in 2005 to investigate the relationship between heat stress and occupational injury among Thai workers. The results provide evidence connecting heat stress and occupational injury in tropical Thailand and also identify several factors that increase heat exposure.

---

[2] A version of Chapter 4 has been published. Tawatsupa B, Yiengprugsawan V, Kjellstrom T, Berecki-Gisolf J, Seubsman S-A, Sleigh A (2013) The association between heat stress and occupational injury among Thai workers: finding of the Thai Cohort Study. *Industrial Health* 51.

Industrial Health 2013, 51, 34–46

Association between Heat Stress and Occupational Injury among Thai Workers: Findings of the Thai Cohort Study

Benjawan TAWATSUPA[1, 2]*, Vasoontara YIENGPRUGSAWAN[2], Tord KJELLSTROM[2, 3], Janneke BERECKI-GISOLF[4], Sam-Ang SEUBSMAN[5] and Adrian SLEIGH[2]

[1] Health Impact Assessment Division, Department of Health, Ministry of Public Health, Thailand
[2] National Centre for Epidemiology and Population Health, ANU College of Medicine, Biology and Environment, Australian National University, Australia
[3] Centre for Global Health Research, Umeå University, Sweden
[4] Monash Injury Research Institute, Monash University, Australia
[5] School of Human Ecology, Sukhothai Thammathirat Open University, Thailand

Received August 24, 2012 and accepted October 24, 2012

Abstract: Global warming will increase heat stress at home and at work. Few studies have addressed the health consequences in tropical low and middle income settings such as Thailand. We report on the association between heat stress and workplace injury among workers enrolled in the large national Thai Cohort Study in 2005 (N=58,495). We used logistic regression to relate heat stress and occupational injury separately for males and females, adjusting for covariate effects of age, income, education, alcohol, smoking, Body Mass Index, job location, job type, sleeping hours, existing illness, and having to work very fast. Nearly 20% of workers experienced occupational heat stress which strongly and significantly associated with occupational injury (adjusted OR 2.12, 95%CI 1.87–2.42 for males and 1.89, 95%CI 1.64–2.18 for females). This study provides evidence connecting heat stress and occupational injury in tropical Thailand and also identifies several factors that increase heat exposure. The findings will be useful for policy makers to consider work-related heat stress problems in tropical Thailand and to develop an occupational health and safety program which is urgently needed given the looming threat of global warming.

Key words: Heat stress, Climate change, Occupational injury, Workers, Thai Cohort Study

Introduction

As global warming proceeds, concern is growing regarding the direct effect of heat stress on human health in many countries[1]. Recently, studies of heat stress have drawn attention to adverse health effects among workers. The international program "High Occupational Temperature: Health and Productivity Suppression" (HOTHAPS)[2] has focused on effects of heat exposure on working people and extended its research to many areas, especially tropical developing countries[3–9].

In low and middle income tropical countries where heat stress is a problem, rapid urbanization and the cash economy may cause workers to do heavy labour for long periods of time under hot and humid conditions, especially those who have low socioeconomic status[10]. As a result, these workers are exposed to excessive heat and are at risk of heat-related illness and increased occupational injury[11].

*To whom correspondence should be addressed.
E-mail: Benjawan.tawatsupa@anu.edu.au

Possible consequences of excessive heat stress include an increase in the likelihood of occupational injury due to fainting, confusion, poor concentration, and psychological distress, resulting in reduced protection and unsafe working conditions. A relationship between heat stress and injury occurrence has been reported several times over the last 35 yr[11-14]. However these studies were conducted in developed non-tropical countries; this leaves unanswered questions about the effect of heat stress on occupational injury in tropical developing countries where temperatures and humidity are already high. In the future, occupational injury risk in all countries could increase as a result of global warming.

Recent reviews have highlighted global warming and health impacts in tropical areas[2, 15]. In Thailand, hot and humid conditions, especially during the hot season (March to June), can be detrimental to population health. The average temperature in Thailand has already increased 0.74°C over the last century[16]. Increasing heat stress is anticipated as Thailand urbanizes, because of the urban heat island effect and progressive global warming[17].

A recent study of workplace occupational heat stress in Thailand by Langkulsen et al.[18] revealed a very serious problem that they classified as "extreme caution" or "danger" in a wide array of work settings. Other studies found that occupational heat stress in Thailand can lead to increased risks of kidney disease and psychological distress[7, 9]. So heat stress is already a public health concern in Thailand and current warming trends are expected to exacerbate the problem due to further increases in air temperatures[19]. However, information on occupational injury related to heat stress in Thailand is still quite limited. As high humidity and hot weather is routine in Thailand, studies on occupational injury almost always overlook heat stress as a contributing factor.

Occupational injury is an important health issue for workers in Thailand[20]. Occupational injury and disease data are recorded primarily through the Workmen's Compensation Fund (WCF) in order to provide cash benefits and medical care to insured workers who suffer workplace injury[21]. In 2008, more than 176,000 cases of occupational injury were reported; 613 cases were fatal and over 45,700 cases reported more than three days absence from work. However, these injury records cover only formal employment which accounts for approximately a third of the Thai workforce[22]. The reports do not capture events at informal work settings, including agricultural work in which heat-related injury is of particular concern due to physically demanding tasks in hot and humid weather[23].

To address the knowledge gap regarding work injury in Thailand, we used the baseline data of a large national adult cohort to examine the epidemiological association between heat stress and injury in the Thai workplace. We identify potential risk factors for heat stress at work. This study will be useful for policy makers considering occupational health and safety program. Such programs are needed to mitigate effects of heat stress at work and prepare for global warming.

Methods

Data and study population

The data derive from the baseline measurements of a large national Thai Cohort Study (TCS) that began in 2005 with distance-learning students enrolled at Sukhothai Thammathirat Open University (STOU). This study investigates the health-risk transition now underway among the Thai population and started with a 20-page mail health questionnaire; details on overall methodology have been reported elsewhere[24]. Overall, 87,134 students aged 15 to 87 yr responded from all areas of Thailand. They represented the adult Thai population well for geographic distribution, income, age and social status[24].

The baseline data included information on health status and on a wide array of socioeconomic characteristics and health behaviours. As well, heat stress at work and occupational injury were recorded. The heat stress and occupational injury questions were in different sections of the questionnaire so answers on these issues were independent of each other. The distribution and frequency of risk factors associated with non-traffic injuries by location have been reported in two recent studies using baseline TCS data[25, 26].

The analysis was restricted to cohort members who reported engaging in paid-work in 2005 (N=62,076). We then excluded 3,581 workers (6%) who did not respond to one or more questions relating to covariates that were potential confounders of heat stress-injury effects (see below). The final analysis group included 58,495 workers (Fig. 1).

Measures of heat stress

The information on individual experiences of heat stress in 2005 was derived from the question: "During the last 12 months, how often did you experience high temperatures which make you uncomfortable?"; respondents answered on a four point scale ("often", "sometimes", "rarely", and "never"). For the main analysis of occupational injury,

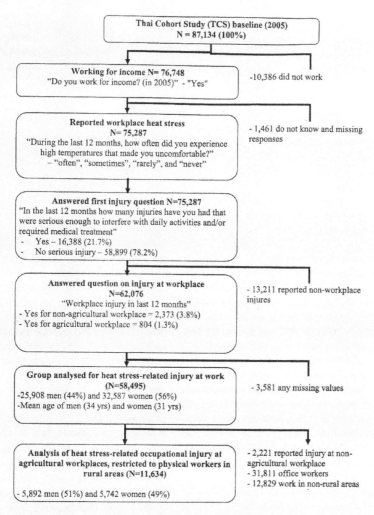

Fig. 1. Selection of the analysed population from the Thai Cohort Study, 2005.

ouped occupational heat stress into three ascending cat-
gories: "never" (rarely + never), "sometimes" and "often".

Measures of occupational injury

Information on occupational injury was based on a
ries of questions as follows. "In the last 12 months how
any serious injuries have you had that were enough to
terfere with daily activities and/or required medical
atment?" with five answer choices (none, once, twice,
ree times, and four times or more). For analysis, injury
quency was dichotomised into "yes/no". If injury was
perienced more than once, respondents reported details
their most serious injury. Injury events were further

characterised by location, identifying occupational injury
as follows: "Where were you when you were seriously
injured?" (home, road, sports facility, workplace (agricultural), workplace (non-agricultural), or other). For our
analyses, "occupational injury" was defined as a serious
injury that occurred in the workplace (agricultural or non-
agricultural). Finally, for workplace injuries respondents
were asked "...how were you seriously injured?" (assault,
fall, other blunt force, drowning, bite/sting, gunshot, stab/
cut, fire/heat, poisoning, and other injury).

Management of confounding

The covariates that could confound heat-injury effects

were initially selected according to our previous experience with heat stress or injury analyses completed for the cohort[7, 9, 26]. Then, separately for males and females, we investigated the relationship of each covariate to the exposure of interest (heat stress) and (separately) to the outcome of interest (occupational injury). Only covariates with statistically significant chi-square tests for both links (ie. to heat stress and to injury) were included as confounders in final multivariable models. The covariates chosen included age, income in Baht/month (US$ 1=40 Baht in 2005), education level, alcohol consumption, smoking, Body Mass Index (using Asian cut-offs for obesity)[27], job location, job type, sleeping hours per day, existing illness in 2005 (heart or kidney disease, stroke or diabetes), and reports of "having to work very fast".

Data processing and statistical analysis

Data scanning and editing were conducted using Thai Scandevet, SQL, and SPSS software. Data analysis used STATA version 12[28]. The main analysis group included 58,495 workers and all epidemiological estimates were made separately for males (25,908) and females (32,587). First, using logistic regression, we calculated crude (bivariate) odds ratios for workplace heat stress and injury. Subsequently, age as a continuous variable was added to the regression model. Then all factors that could confound workplace heat stress effects on occupational injury (see above) were included as covariates in the multivariable logistic regression analyses. These produced fully adjusted odds ratios, 95% confidence limits, and p-trends showing the dose-response of heat stress effects on occupational injury for males and females.

To test for modification of the heat stress effects, for males and females, we constructed a figure showing covariate-stratified analyses of heat stress-occupational injury relationships. We included all covariates that had statistically significant relationships with both heat stress and occupational injury. These sex-covariate-stratified heat stress-injury odds ratios were adjusted for the mutual effects of all the covariates.

Finally, we examined the association between heat stress and occupational injury among agricultural workers in Thailand. We restricted analysis to the 11,634 cohort members who worked in physical jobs in rural areas having excluded those who reported injury at non-agricultural workplaces.

Ethical considerations

Ethical approval was obtained from Sukhothai Tham-

mathirat Open University Research and Developm Institute (protocol 0522/10) and the Australian Natic University Human Research Ethics Committee (proto 2004344 and 2009570). Informed, written consent obtained from all participants.

Results

Characteristics of the cohort

Among the 58,495 Thai baseline (2005) cohort me bers who worked for income, 25,908 (44%) were m and 32,587 were female (Table 1). Overall, 70% of cohort was aged between 15–34 yr with the average ag females below that of males (31 vs 34 yr). Half the ma and 39% of females had education at high school le 28% of males and 41% of females had low incomes (≤7, Bt/month). Males were more likely to work in rural ar (47% vs 44%) and more likely to have physical jobs (ski and manual) (50% vs 40%). Among working ma 11% reported that they were regular alcohol drinkers 20% were current smokers, which was much higher t females (only 0.6% of females reported being regu drinkers and 0.9% reported being current smokers). Ma were more likely to be obese than females (24% vs 10 On average, 12% of workers slept less than 6 h per ni and 52% often had to work very fast.

Heat stress at work and occupational injury

Overall, 18% (N=10,784) of the analysed group 58,495 workers reported that they often experienc uncomfortably high temperatures at work (Table 2). T occurred more often among males than females (22% 16%). Females reported never/rarely experiencing h stress at work more frequently than males (56% vs 44 Further analyses for heat-related injury at work are d separately for males and females.

Serious injury at work over the previous year was ported by 5% of the whole cohort in 2005 (Table 2). It higher among males than females (7% vs 4%). The type occupational injury was heterogeneous but the most co mon categories were "blunt force" (24%), "stab-cut" (21 "fall" (18%), and "other" (29%); females were more lik to fall and males were more likely to experience stab- or blunt force injury (Table 2).

Association of cohort attributes with workplace heat str

Figure 2 summarises the association of cohort cova ates with heat stress, the exposure of interest, for male a female workers. The crude (bivariate) age association w

Table 1. Socioeconomic status, health behaviour, and other characteristics in a national cohort of 58,495 workers in Thailand

Cohort attributes	Men		Women		Total	
	N	%	N	%	N	%
Total	25,908	44.3	32,587	55.7	58,495	100.0
Age group (yr)						
Less than 35	16,199	62.5	24,771	76.0	40,970	70.0
≥35	9709	37.5	7816	24.0	17,525	30.0
Education						
University	6,349	24.5	9,034	27.7	15,383	26.3
Diploma	6,369	24.6	10,830	33.2	17,199	29.4
High school	13,190	50.9	12,723	39.0	25,913	44.3
Personal income (Baht/month)[a]						
20,001+	4,020	15.5	3,012	9.2	7,032	12.0
10,001–20,000	8,231	31.8	7,779	23.9	16,010	27.4
7,001–10,000	6,422	24.8	8,615	26.4	15,037	25.7
≤7,000	7,235	27.9	13,181	40.5	20,416	34.9
Alcohol consumption						
Never	2,493	9.6	12,809	39.3	15,302	26.2
Stopped/Occasional drinker	20,688	79.9	19,571	60.1	40,259	68.8
Regular drinker	2,727	10.5	207	0.6	2,934	5.0
Smoking						
Never smoked	12,993	50.2	31,140	95.6	44,133	75.5
Ex-smoker	7,745	29.9	1,149	3.5	8,894	15.2
Current smoker	5,170	20.0	298	0.9	5,468	9.4
BMI in 2005						
Normal weight (18.5 to <23)	12,565	48.5	19,497	59.8	32,062	54.8
Underweight (<18.5)	1,375	5.3	6,617	20.3	7,992	13.7
Overweight (23 to <25)	5,856	22.6	3,196	9.8	9,052	15.5
Obese (≥25)	6,112	23.6	3,277	10.1	9,389	16.1
Job location						
Bangkok	3,905	15.1	6,543	20.1	10,448	17.9
Urban	9,859	38.1	11,847	36.4	21,706	37.1
Rural	12,144	46.9	14,197	43.6	26,341	45.0
Job type						
Office job	13,097	50.6	19,698	60.5	32,795	56.1
Physical job	12,811	49.5	12,889	39.6	25,700	43.9
Sleeping hours per day						
6–8 hr	20,013	77.3	24,574	75.4	44,587	76.2
>8 hr	2,829	10.9	3,879	11.9	6,708	11.5
<6 hr	3,066	11.8	4,134	12.7	7,200	12.3
Existing illness[b]						
No other disease	24,854	95.9	31,529	96.7	56,383	96.4
have existing illness	1,054	4.1	1,058	3.3	2,112	3.6
Have to work very fast						
Rarely/never	1,946	7.5	2,070	6.4	4016	6.9
Sometime	11,301	43.6	12,802	39.3	24103	41.2
Often	12,661	48.9	17,715	54.4	30376	51.9

[a]US$ 1 = 40 Baht in 2005, [b]Existing illness in 2005 = people report doctor-diagnosed heart or kidney disease, stroke or diabetes.

Table 2. Reported heat stress at work and occupational injury in a national cohort of 58,495 workers in Thailand

Heat stress and occupational injury	Males		Females		Total	
	N	%	N	%	N	%
Total	25,908	44.3	32,587	55.7	58,495	100.0
Heat stress						
Rarely /Never	11,260	43.5	18,125	55.6	29,385	50.2
Sometimes	8,899	34.4	9,427	28.9	18,326	31.3
Often	5,749	22.2	5,035	15.5	10,784	18.4
Serious injury at work						
No serious injury	24,236	93.6	31,299	96.1	55,535	94.9
Occupational injury	1,672	6.5	1,288	4	2,960	5.1
Type of occupational injury						
Other blunt force	400	25.5	262	21.2	662	23.6
Stab-cut	371	23.7	215	17.4	586	20.9
Fall (not pushed)	228	14.6	271	21.9	499	17.8
Bite-sting (animal, insect)	110	7.0	105	8.5	215	7.7
Road traffic injury	141	8.4	73	5.7	214	7.7
Fire-heat	59	3.8	43	3.5	102	7.2
Poisoning	52	3.3	32	2.6	84	3.6
Assault (punch, push or kick)	33	2.1	9	0.7	42	3.0
Drowning	5	0.3	5	0.4	10	1.5
Gun shot	5	0.3	2	0.2	7	0.4
Other injury	405	25.9	402	32.5	807	28.8

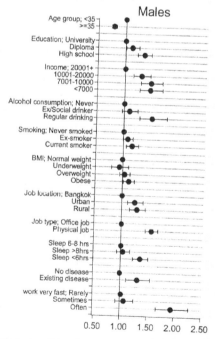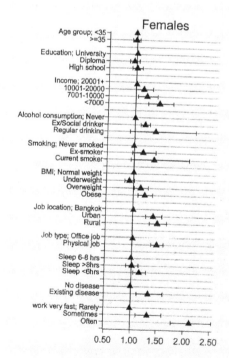

Fig. 2. Association of cohort covariates with heat stress[a].

[a]Workplace heat stress as dependent variable (often/not often); age group ORs (95% CI) not adjusted; all other covariate ORs mutually adjusted (with age included as a continuous variable).

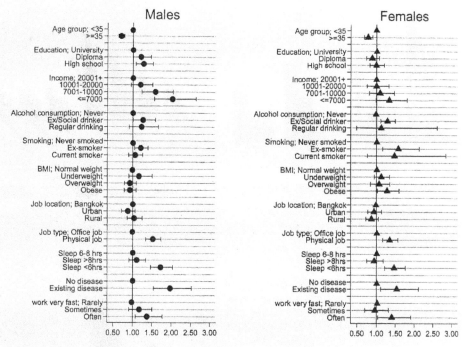

Fig. 3. Association of cohort covariates with occupational injury[a].

[a]Occupational injury as dependent variable (yes/no); age group ORs (95% CI) not adjusted; for all other covariate ORs mutually adjusted (with age included as a continuous variable).

at stress is shown with age divided into two groups; all e other variables tested for their association with heat ress are adjusted for age as a continuous variable and utually adjusted for other covariates. For both sexes, all variates significantly associated with occupational heat ess (except age group and education level in females). ccupational heat stress was notably higher for those with wer income, regular drinking, current smoking, obesity, eeping less than six hours per day, having "existing ill-ss", and often "having to work very fast". Workers in ysical jobs had much more heat stress at work than did ice workers ($p<0.001$). Those who worked in rural areas ore frequently reported heat stress at work than workers urban area or Bangkok ($p<0.001$).

sociation of cohort attributes with occupational injury

The odds of occupational injury reduced significantly h age for both sexes ($p<0.001$) (Fig. 3). Risks of occu-tional injury were higher among those with low income, rking in physical jobs, sleeping less than 6 h per day, ving "existing illness", and often "having to work very

fast". Most of these associations were significant and the pattern for males and females were similar; however, in-come and education effects were more extreme for males.

Association of heat stress and occupational injury by age, income and job type

Overall, the association of heat stress with occupational injury is worse for males than females. It was especially notable for younger workers aged less than 35 yr (Fig. 4). Among males less than 35 yr old (Fig. 4), with low income (≤7,000 Bt/month) (Fig. 5), and with physical jobs (Fig. 6) the proportion reporting injury over the previous 12 months exceeded 10%.

Effects of heat stress on occupational injury

Occupational injury was reported by 10% of males who were often exposed to workplace heat stress compared to 4% who were never exposed. For females, occupational injury affected 7% who were often exposed to heat stress compared to 3% who were never exposed (Table 3). For both males and females the crude ORs linking heat stress

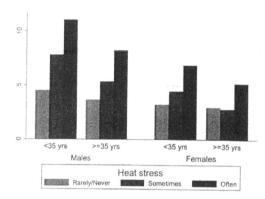

Fig. 4. Occupational injury (%)* by heat stress, sex and age.
*Proportion of Thai workers reporting injury over previous 12 months (see methods).

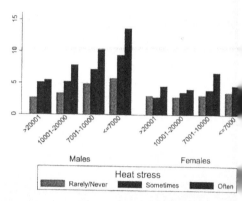

Fig. 5. Occupational injury (%)* by heat stress, sex and income
*Proportion of Thai workers reporting injury over previous 12 mc (see methods).

and occupational injury showed a strong association (OR > 2) and a notable dose response. Age group adjustment had little effect. The fully adjusted ORs derived from models that included continuous age (yrs), income, education, job location, smoking, alcohol drinking, BMI, job location, job type, sleeping hours, existing disease, and having to work very fast. The covariate-adjusted dose-response relationships of heat stress and occupational injury remained strong and significant for both sexes (adjusted OR for heat stress "often" 2.12 (males) and 1.90 (females), p-trend<0.001).

Modification of the heat stress-injury effects was investigated using stratified analyses for each of the significant covariates (Fig. 7). For each covariate, heat stress-injury OR analyses were restricted in strata corresponding to each value of the covariate. For most of these covariates, there was little evidence that their values modified the heat stress-injury ORs. But, for both sexes, heat stress-injury effects were modified by a few covariates: the ORs substantially increased for low education level, regular drinking, short sleeping hours, and having to work fast.

Effects of heat stress on occupational injury in agricultural workplaces

Finally, we explored effects of heat stress on occupational injury that occurred in the agriculture workplace by restricting analysis to those respondents who worked in rural areas with physical jobs, excluding those who reported injury at non-agricultural workplaces. Overall, 23% of physical workers in rural areas often experienced heat stress – 27% for males and 19% for females (data not

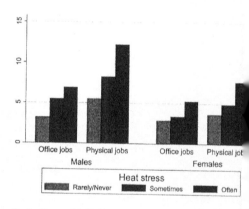

Fig. 6. Occupational injury (%)* by heat stress, sex and job typ
*Proportion of Thai workers reporting injury over previous 12 mc (see methods).

shown). Heat stress in this restricted rural physical j group is higher than among the 58,459 working col members, for whom the overall rate was 18% (Table 2).

The pattern linking heat stress and occupational inj at agricultural workplaces in Table 4 was similar to t shown for workers in Table 3. Male physical work reported 228 occupational injuries at agricultural wo places; these injuries affected 6% of those often expos to heat stress compared to 3% of those unexposed (adjus OR=1.99). Female physical workers reported 84 occu tional injuries at agricultural workplaces; these injur affected 3% of those often heat stressed at work compa to 1% of the unexposed (adjusted OR=2.58).

Table 3. Associations between heat stress and occupational injury among male and female workers (N=58,495)

Heat stress 2005		Occupational Injury		Odds Ratios (ORs)				
		N	%	Crude	Age adj.[a]	Adj.[b]	(95% CI)	p-trend
Male	N = 25,908	1,672	6.5					
	Never/Rarely	473	4.2	1	1	1		<0.001
	Sometimes	616	6.9	1.70***	1.68***	1.54***	(1.36–1.74)	
	Often	583	10.1	2.57***	2.51***	2.12***	(1.87–2.42)	
Females	N = 32,587	1,288	4					
	Never/Rarely	578	3.2	1	1	1		<0.001
	Sometimes	384	4.1	1.29***	1.30***	1.24***	(1.08–1.42)	
	Often	326	6.5	2.10***	2.11***	1.90***	(1.64–2.18)	

*p-value<0.05, **p-value<0.01, ***p-value<0.001.

[a] Associations of heat stress and occupational injury expressed as ORs adjusted for age (<35 yr, ≥35 yr).

[b] Associations of heat stress and occupational injury expressed as ORs adjusted for age (yr), alcohol, smoking, BMI, income, education, job type, job location, sleeping hours, having to work very fast, and existing illness (see Methods).

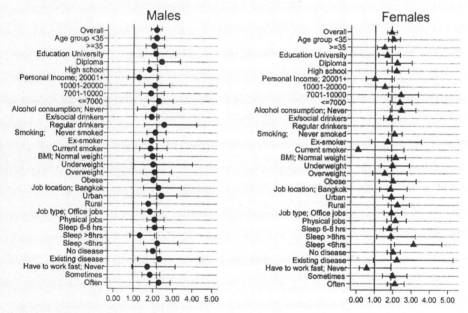

Fig. 7. Stratified analyses of the association between heat stress and occupational injury for males and females[a].

[a] Analyses of heat stress-injury odds ratios (ORs) are repeated for each value of each covariate; all these stratified ORs (95% CI) are mutually adjusted for the influence of all other covariates.

Discussion

Principal findings

Heat stress at work in Thailand has a strong and significant association with occupational injury. This is important because occupational heat stress affected nearly 20% of Thai workers in the national cohort. These findings add to the limited literature on the association between heat stress and occupational injury of Thai workers. The associa-

tion between heat stress at work and occupational injury remained substantial and statistically significant after accounting for the effects of age, income, education, alcohol, smoking, Body Mass Index, job location, job type, sleeping hours per day, existing illness in 2005, and having to work very fast. For rural physical workers at agriculture workplaces we found a similar association between heat stress and occupational injury.

Table 4. Associations between heat stress and occupational injury at agricultural workplaces among male and female workers in rural areas with physical jobs (N=11,634)

Heat stress 2005		Occupational injury		ORs				
		N	%	Crude	Age adj.[a]	Adj.[b]	(95%CI)	p-trend
Males	N=5,892	228	3.9					
	Never/Rarely	59	2.8	1	1	1		<0.001
	Sometimes	81	3.7	1.35	1.35	1.31	(0.93–1.85)	
	Often	88	5.6	2.09***	2.08***	1.99***	(1.41–2.81)	
Females	N=5,742	84	1.5					
	Never/Rarely	25	0.9	1	1	1		0.001
	Sometimes	31	1.6	1.78*	1.74*	1.64	(0.96–2.80)	
	Often	28	2.5	2.80***	2.74***	2.58***	(1.49–4.47)	

*p-value<0.05, **p-value<0.01, ***p-value<0.001.

[a]Associations of heat stress and occupational injury expressed as ORs adjusted for age (<35 yr, ≥35 yr)

[b]Associations of heat stress and occupational injury expressed as ORs adjusted for age (yrs), alcohol, smoking, BMI, income, education, job type, job location, sleeping hours, having to work very fast, and existing illness (see Methods).

Strengths and weakness of the study

The main advantage of this study is that it was based on a large national cohort of 58,495 workers who represent well working age Thais for geographic location, demographic attributes and socioeconomic status. Cohort members are better educated than average Thais of the same age and sex[24]. Because of their education advantage, workplace heat stress exposure in the cohort may under-represent the magnitude of the problem in the general population. Although this impacts the reported exposure (which was already substantial with 20% of the Thai cohort workers experiencing occupational heat stress) it is unlikely to affect the reported associations between exposures and outcomes.

The cohort data have a wide range of values for variables of interest, revealing the relationship between heat stress and occupational injury. We strengthened our results by the restricted analysis of 11,634 workers with physical jobs in rural areas, excluding those reporting injury in the non-agricultural workplaces. The patterns of the association between heat stress and occupational injury were similar to the overall analysis of 58,459 cohort workers.

A limitation of this study could have arisen if people had experienced their heat stress during a hot period and their injury during a cold period. If this happened the frequency of injury and the frequency of heat stress would be unrelated. However, there is no really cold period in most of Thailand and our data showed a consistent association between reported heat stress and reported injury over the previous 12 months. But we cannot prove that the injury occurred at the same time as the heat stress and such a linked measurement was not a feasible part our study

design. We can prove the association we found is un to be due to chance (p<0.001) and this fits well wi epidemiological model linking heat stress to increase jury risk. The heat-injury model is supported by a dos sponse whereby more heat stress associated with incr odds of injury.

The main disadvantage of this study is that it coul directly establish that the occupational injury arose result of heat stress. There are some difficulties in preting causality between heat stress and occupation jury given that we cannot formally be sure that heat preceded occupational injury. However, it is not l that heat stress resulted from injury as there is no ob mechanism for such an effect.

Another problem is the unknown source or nature c heat stress at work as this was not reported in the c data. Furthermore, we were not able to make direct surements of work environments or occupational inju we classify this study as preliminary in nature.

Compare with other studies

Occupational heat stress is a problem in Thail especially in agriculture workplaces[18, 29]. Our study found that Thais often work under heat stress, espec those with physical jobs in rural areas. The proportic workers in both sexes who reported occupational ir declined with age; this may reflect ageing, working ex ence, and shifting away from work with high risk o jury[30]. The younger age group reported more occupati injury perhaps because of their lower socioecono status. They cannot afford to go to a regular university are more likely to have a job with less safety[14].

As expected from other studies, we found a higher risk of serious occupational injury among males[30, 31]. Another important risk factor significantly associated with occupational injury was low income ($\leq$7,000 Baht/month), already noted with a previous study of the Thai cohort on risk factors associated with injury[26]. As with other studies on occupational injury, we found that the risk of injury related to job type, rural job location[32], and frequency of alcohol consumption[33].

Other TCS studies reported associations between occupational heat stress and adverse health outcomes, including poor self-assessed overall health, psychological distress, and incident kidney disease among Thai workers[7, 9]. This study now adds additional concerns about the effects of heat stress on occupational injury in Thailand.

Significance of this study

The findings support the reported by Kjellstrom *et al.*[2] that occupational heat stress increases the risk of serious injury and ill-health among workers who are exposed to hot and humid work environments, especially in low income-tropical countries[4]. The combination of hot weather and high humidity together with workers' physical exertion and dehydration can cause potentially heat-related illness or heat exhaustion (fainting or collapse) which could increase occupational injury and associated costs as well as reduce work performance and productivity.

Moreover, heat-stress related occupational injuries are especially important at present because we can expect that the existing heat stress problem will worsen if global warming continues and workplaces become even more thermally stressful[34]. Given the constrained resources in middle-income Thailand and the lack of effective policy and guidelines on prevention and management of heat stress and occupational injury, our results on occupational injury are of particular concern.

In Thailand, a large proportion of the population is in the working age group. Furthermore, the National Statistical Office reported that 46% of employed Thais were working in the agricultural sector[35]. As already shown in the final analysis of this study, physical workers in rural areas often worked under heat stress.

Thai workers must take safety precautions while working under heat stress and policymakers should develop the interventions to prevent occupational injury, especially during summer for the new young workers. Prevention of heat stress-related injury through education, training and procedures is needed to protect workers in all type of work environments.

Future research

We have used telephone contact to validate the occurrence of heat stress for 82% of a random sample of 135 cohort members who had self-reported heat stress (data not shown). The validation boosts our confidence in the self-reported measurement of heat exposure. We also queried the source of the heat and discovered that it often came from the prevailing external air temperature when working outdoors (48%), from the work process itself (31%), from working indoors without air conditioning (13%), or from working in a hot vehicle (6%). Now direct observations of heat stress and its effects in informative work settings are needed to add information on the physical and biomechanical mechanisms generating heat stress and linking it to injury and other adverse health effects.

Also, we need to investigate heat stress-related injury so we can accurately characterize associated occupational injury. As well, we should investigate heat-related injury in different regions of Thailand because the geography and heat stress are different. For example, in Thailand temperatures vary considerably during the day and night in the North and vary little in the South.

Conclusion

The association between occupational heat stress and occupational injury reported here is a great concern. More information is needed on the nature and source of the heat stress and on the associated injury. Continued urbanisation and global warming will make these trends worse for workers in tropical developing countries like Thailand. Injury interventions in such settings need to include strategies that mitigate occupational heat stress. Also we need to develop and test interventions that reduce the number and severity of occupational injuries in Thailand.

Conflicts of interest

The authors declare that we have no competing interests.

Acknowledgements

This study was supported by the International Collaborative Research Grants Scheme with joint grants from the Wellcome Trust UK (GR071587MA) and the Australian National Health and Medical Research Council (NHMRC 268055), and as a global health grant from the NHMRC (585426). These funding bodies play no role in the preparation or submission of this manuscript. We thank the Thai Cohort Study team*, the staff at Sukhothai Thammathirat Open University (STOU) who assisted with student contact, and the STOU students who are participating in the cohort study. We also thank Dr Bandit Thinkamrop and his team from Khon Kaen University for guiding us successfully through the complex data processing.

*Thai Cohort Study Team

Thailand: Jaruwan Chokhanapitak, Suttanit Hounthasarn, Suwanee Khamman, Daoruang Pandee, Suttinan Pangsap, Tippawan Prapamontol, Janya Puengson, Sam-ang Seubsman, Boonchai Somboonsook, Nintita Sripaiboonkij, Pathumvadee Somsamai, Duangkae Vilainerun, Wanee Wimonwattanaphan, Cha-aim Pachanee, Arunrat Tangmunkongvorakul, Benjawan Tawatsupa, Wimalin Rimpeekool

Australia: Chris Bain, Emily Banks, Cathy Banwell, Bruce Caldwell, Gordon Carmichael, Tarie Dellora, Jane Dixon, Sharon Friel, David Harley, Matthew Kelly, Tord Kjellstrom, Lynette Lim, Anthony McMichael, Tanya Mark, Adrian Sleigh, Lyndall Strazdins, Vasoontara Yiengprugsawan, Susan Jordan, Janneke Berecki-Gisolf, Rod McClure

References

1) Confalonieri U, Menne B, Akhtar R, Ebi K, Hauengue M, Kovats RS, Revich B, Woodward A (2007) Human Health. Climate change 2007: Impacts, adaptation and vulnerability, contribution of working group II to the fourth assessment report of the Intergovernmental Panel on Climate Change. Cambridge University Press. http://www.ipcc-wg2.org. Accessed March 13, 2012.

2) Kjellstrom T, Gabrysch S, Lemke B, Dear K (2009) The "Hothaps" program for assessing climate change impacts on occupational health and productivity: an invitation to carry out field studies. Glob Health Action 2, 2.

3) Kjellstrom T (2009) Climate change, direct heat exposure, health and well-being in low and middle-income countries. Glob Health Action 2, 1–3. [Medline]

4) Kjellstrom T, Holmér I, Lemke B (2009) Workplace heat stress, health and productivity – an increasing challenge for low and middle-income countries during climate change. Global Health Action 2.

5) Hyatt OM, Lemke B, Kjellstrom T (2010) Regional maps of occupational heat exposure: past, present, and potential future. Global Health Action 3.

6) Mathee A, Oba J, Rose A (2010) Climate change impacts on working people (the HOTHAPS initiative): findings of the South African pilot study. Global Health Action 3.

7) Tawatsupa B, Lim LL-Y, Kjellstrom T, Seubsman S, S A, the Thai Cohort Study team (2010) The associ between overall health, psychological distress, occupational heat stress among a large national coho 40,913 Thai workers. Global Health Action 3.

8) Kjellstrom T, Crowe J (2011) Climate change, work heat exposure, and occupational health and productiv Central America. Int J Occup Environ Health 17, 270 [Medline] [CrossRef]

9) Tawatsupa B, Lim LL-Y, Kjellstrom T, Seubsman S, S A, the Thai Cohort Study team (2012) Association bet occupational heat stress and kidney disease among 3 workers in the Thai Cohort Study (TCS). J Epidemic 251. [Medline]

10) McMichael AJ (2000) The urban environment and hea a world of increasing globalization: issues for devele countries. Bull World Health Organ 78, 1117–26. [Me

11) Cho KS, Lee SH (1978) Occupational health haz of mine workers. Bull World Health Organ 56, 20: [Medline]

12) Enander AE, Hygge S (1990) Thermal stress and h performance. Scand J Work Environ Health 16 (Sup 44–50. [Medline] [CrossRef]

13) Morabito M, Cecchi L, Crisci A, Modesti PA, Orla S (2006) Relationship between work-related acci and hot weather conditions in Tuscany (Central Italy Health 44, 458–64. [Medline] [CrossRef]

14) Fogleman M, Fakhrzadeh L, Bernard TE (2005) relationship between outdoor thermal conditions and injury in an aluminum smelter. Int J Ind Ergon 35, 4 [CrossRef]

15) McMichael AJ, Patz J, Kovats RS (1998) Impacts of g environmental change on future health and health ca tropical countries. Br Med Bull 54, 475–88. [Med [CrossRef]

16) Limsakul A, Limjirakan S, Sriburi T (2009) Trends in temperature extremes in Thailand. Ministry of Na Resources and Environment, Second National Confer on Natural Resources and Environment Bangkok, Thai 59.

17) Taniguchi M (2006) Anthropogenic effects on subsu temperature in Bangkok. Clim Past Discuss 2, 831 [CrossRef]

18) Langkulsen U, Vichit-Vadakan N, Taptagaporn S (2 Health impact of climate change on occupational health productivity in Thailand. Global Health Action 3.

19) Thai Meteorological Department (2007) Climate ch in Thailand for last 52 years. Meteorological Departr Thailand. http://www.tmd.go.th/info/info.php?FileID Accessed July 4, 2010.

20) Siriruttanapruk S, Anantagunathi P (2004) Occupati health and safety situation and research priority in Thai Ind Health 42, 135–40. [Medline] [CrossRef]

21) Choi BCK (1996) Recording, notification, compila

and classification of statistics of occupational accidents and diseases: the thai experience. J Occup Environ Med **38**, 1151–60. [Medline] [CrossRef]

22) Institute for Population and Social Research (2010) Thai health. 12 health indicators of Thailand's workforce. Mahidol University, Bangkok.

23) Hansen E, Donohoe M (2003) Health issues of migrant and seasonal farmworkers. J Health Care Poor Underserved **14**, 153–64. [Medline]

24) Sleigh AC, Seubsman S Bain C, Thai Cohort Team (2008) Cohort profile: the Thai cohort of 87,134 open university students. Int J Epidemiol **37**, 266–72. [Medline] [CrossRef]

25) Stephan K, McClure R, Seubsman SA, Kelly M, Yiengprugsawan V, Bain C, Sleigh A (2010) Review of injuries over a one year period among 87,134 adults studying at an open university in Thailand. Southeast Asian J Trop Med Public Health **41**, 1220–30. [Medline]

26) Yiengprugsawan V, Stephan K, McClure R, Kelly M, Seubsman S, Bain C, Sleigh AC (2012) Risk factors for injury in a national cohort of 87,134 Thai adults. Public Health **126**, 33–9. [Medline] [CrossRef]

27) Kanazawa M, Yoshiike N, Osaka T, Numba Y, Zimmet P, Inoue S (2002) Criteria and classification of obesity in Japan and Asia-Oceania. Asia Pac J Clin Nutr **11**, S732–7. [Medline] [CrossRef]

28) StataCorp (2011) Stata 12.0 for Windows. StataCorporation, College Station TX.

29) Jakreng C (2010) Physical health effects from occupational exposure to natural heat among salt production workers in Samutsonghram province. Srinakharinwirot university, Bangkok.

30) Curtis Breslin F, Polzer J, MacEachen E, Morrongiello B, Shannon H (2007) Workplace injury or "part of the job"?: Towards a gendered understanding of injuries and complaints among young workers. Soc Sci Med **64**, 782–93. [Medline] [CrossRef]

31) Fan J, McLeod CB, Koehoorn M (2012) Descriptive epidemiology of serious work-related injuries in British Columbia, Canada. PLoS ONE **7**, e38750. [Medline] [CrossRef]

32) Dembe AE, Erickson JB, Delbos R (2004) Predictors of work-related injuries and illnesses: national survey findings. J Occup Environ Hyg **1**, 542–50. [Medline] [CrossRef]

33) Dawson DA (1994) Heavy drinking and the risk of occupational injury. Accid Anal Prev **26**, 655–65. [Medline] [CrossRef]

34) Kjellstrom T, Kovats RS, Lloyd SJ, Holt T, Tol RS (2009) The direct impact of climate change on regional labor productivity. Arch Environ Occup Health **64**, 217–27. [Medline] [CrossRef]

35) National Statistical Office (2008) Key statistics of Thailand 2008. Ministry of Information and Communication Technology, Thailand. http://service.nso.go.th/nso/thailand/dataFile/23/J23W/J23W/th/0.htm. Accessed May 25, 2009.

CHAPTER 5: HEAT STRESS AND KIDNEY DISEASE[3]

Occupational heat stress is a well-known problem, particularly in tropical countries, affecting workers' health status. One interesting feature of the health status of Thai workers in a large national Thai Cohort Study (TCS) and in the general population is a recent increase of incident kidney disease. Kidney disease has been reported to be related to heat stress in some studies but there are only a few reports in tropical and developing countries. Fortunately, TCS data are available to investigate the heat stress exposure at baseline in 2005, and also prolonged heat stress exposure in the follow-up study in 2009. Thus, this chapter presents a longitudinal study of the relationship between self-reported occupational heat stress and incidence of self-reported doctor-diagnosed kidney disease among Thai workers.

[3] A version of Chapter 5 has been published. Tawatsupa B, Lim LL-Y, Kjellstrom T, Seubsman S, Sleigh A, the Thai Cohort Study team (2012) Association between occupational heat stress and kidney disease among 37,816 workers in the Thai Cohort Study (TCS). *Journal of Epidemiology* 22:251-260. DOI: 10.2188/jea.JE20110082

J Epidemiol 2012;22(3):251-2●
doi:10.2188/jea.JE201100●

Original Article

Association Between Occupational Heat Stress and Kidney Disease Among 37 816 Workers in the Thai Cohort Study (TCS)

Benjawan Tawatsupa[1,2], Lynette L-Y Lim[2], Tord Kjellstrom[2,3], Sam-ang Seubsman[2,4], Adrian Sleigh[2], and the Thai Cohort Study Team*

[1]Health Impact Assessment Division, Department of Health, Ministry of Public Health, Nonthaburi, Thailand
[2]National Centre for Epidemiology and Population Health, The Australian National University, Canberra ACT, Australia
[3]Centre for Global Health Research, Umeå University, Umeå, Sweden
[4]Thai Health-Risk Transition: National Cohort Study, School of Human Ecology, Sukhothai Thammathirat Open University, Nonthaburi, Thailand

Received August 4, 2011; accepted December 5, 2011; released online February 18, 2012

ABSTRACT

Background: We examined the relationship between self-reported occupational heat stress and incidence of self-reported doctor-diagnosed kidney disease in Thai workers.

Methods: Data were derived from baseline (2005) and follow-up (2009) self-report questionnaires from a large national Thai Cohort Study (TCS). Analysis was restricted to full-time workers ($n = 17\,402$ men and 20 414 women) without known kidney disease at baseline. We used logistic regression models to examine the association of incident kidney disease with heat stress at work, after adjustment for smoking, alcohol drinking, body mass index, and a large number of socioeconomic and demographic characteristics.

Results: Exposure to heat stress was more common in men than in women (22% vs 15%). A significant association between heat stress and incident kidney disease was observed in men (adjusted odds ratio [OR] = 1.48, 95% CI: 1.01–2.16). The risk of kidney disease was higher among workers reporting workplace heat stress in both 2005 and 2009. Among men exposed to prolonged heat stress, the odds of developing kidney disease was 2.22 times that of men without such exposure (95% CI 1.48–3.35, P-trend <0.001). The incidence of kidney disease was even higher among men aged 35 years or older in a physical job: 2.2% exposed to prolonged heat stress developed kidney disease compared with 0.4% with no heat exposure (adjusted OR = 5.30, 95% CI 1.17–24.13).

Conclusions: There is an association between self-reported occupational heat stress and self-reported doctor-diagnosed kidney disease in Thailand. The results indicate a need for occupational health interventions for heat stress among workers in tropical climates.

Key words: occupational heat stress; kidney disease; Thai Cohort Study; Thailand

INTRODUCTION

The rising frequency of very hot days and the spread of urban heat-island effects in many cities are affecting the health of elderly populations.[1] Working people are also affected by heat stress, especially outdoor workers exposed to excessive heat because of their job.[1] Health impacts from elevated air temperature have been observed in many studies, and respiratory, cardiovascular, and kidney disease have all been linked to global warming.[1-4] Moreover, occupational heat stress was found to be associated with worse mental hea● and psychological distress in Thailand.[5]

The body's natural methods of cooling include convecti● conduction, and evaporation of sweat. Only evaporation ● lower body temperature when air temperature is higher t● 35°C (which is common in tropical countries), and it is ● effective when humidity is high.[6] Evaporation leads to loss● body water and electrolytes, especially sodium and chlori● which are responsible for maintenance of overall fl● balance. Depletion of water and sodium results in loss●

Address for correspondence. Benjawan Tawatsupa, National Centre for Epidemiology and Population Health, The Australian National University, Canberra A● Australia (e-mail: benjawan.tawatsupa@anu.edu.au).
*Thai Cohort Study Team: Thailand—Jaruwan Chokhanapitak, Chaiyun Churewong, Suttanit Hounthasarn, Suwanee Khamman, Daoruang Pandee, Sut● Pangsap, Tippawan Prapamontol, Janya Puengson, Yodyiam Sangrattanakul, Sam-ang Seubsman, Boonchai Somboonsook, Nintita Sripaiboonkij, Pathumv● Somsamai, Duangkae Vilainerun, Wanee Wimonwattanaphan; Australia—Chris Bain, Emily Banks, Cathy Banwell, Bruce Caldwell, Gordon Carmichael, ● Dellora, Jane Dixon, Sharon Friel, David Harley, Matthew Kelly, Tord Kjellstrom, Lynette Lim, Roderick McClure, Anthony McMichael, Tanya Mark, A● Sleigh, Lyndall Strazdins, Vasoontara Yiengprugsawan.

extracellular fluid volume, which can place acute or chronic stress on kidney function and ultimately lead to kidney disease.[7]

Kidney disease is usually divided into 2 forms: acute kidney failure (sudden loss of kidney function) and chronic kidney failure (slow, gradual loss of kidney function). Acute kidney failure can result from severe dehydration. Slow loss of kidney function is exacerbated by diabetes, hypertension, and blockage from kidney stones. Kidney stones are more common with chronic dehydration.[8] Heat waves and related dehydration are associated with both acute renal failure and chronic renal disease.[2,4,9–11]

In Thailand, kidney disease is a major cause of death among middle-aged adults. The number of deaths from renal failure has increased from 8895 in 2001 to 11 246 in 2005 and 2 195 in 2007.[12] A high incidence of urolithiasis (kidney stones) with a male/female ratio of 1.6 to 2 was observed among manual workers (farmers, laborers, housekeepers), especially farmers.[13,14] The increase in renal deaths and high incidence of urolithiasis in manual workers are worrisome because they might be partially caused by increasing heat stress in a hot, humid country with dynamic economic development. From 1951 to 2003, the mean maximum daily temperature in Thailand increased by 0.56°C, and the mean minimum temperature increased even more, by 1.44°C.[15] Increasing heat stress is anticipated as Thailand urbanizes, due to the urban heat-island effect and the continuing increase in average temperature associated with global warming.

A related issue is the effect of occupational heat stress, especially in tropical countries, where temperatures and other climate variables are already thermally stressful.[16] Problems regarding heat exposure in occupational settings exist in Thailand,[17] but there are no studies of heat-related kidney disease. This study examines the association between occupational exposure to heat stress and kidney disease. The data are derived from the self-reports of a large national cohort of Thai distance learning students of Open University whose social and physical environment and health outcomes have been followed from 2005 to 2009.[18]

METHODS

The Thai Cohort Study (TCS) is an ongoing examination of the health-risk transition in the adult Thai population. At baseline in 2005, all cohort members were enrolled as distance learning students at Sukhothai Thammathirat Open University (STOU), resided all over Thailand, lived with their families, and worked part- or full-time. The study started with a 2005 mailed baseline questionnaire that inquired about sociodemographic variables, work, health and injuries, social networks and well-being, diet and physical activity, tobacco, alcohol, and transport. A follow-up questionnaire in 2009 repeated some of the sociodemographic and occupational measurements and obtained information on heat stress and

other work hazards, well being, mental health, self-rated health, and information on specific diseases, including kidney disease. There were 87 134 respondents at baseline, and 70% (60 569) responded to the follow-up study. Those who were included in the 2009 follow-up were the same persons as those studied in 2005, and the 2 data sets have been linked.[18–20]

Occupational heat stress in 2005 was assessed by the question: "During the last 12 months, how often did you experience high temperatures that made you uncomfortable at work? (in 2005)", to which respondents answered on a 4-point scale: often, sometimes, rarely, and never. For analysis of 2005 heat stress, the scale was collapsed to 3 categories by combining rarely and never. Heat stress in 2009 was evaluated using the question: "How often did the hot period this year interfere with your work? (in 2009)", to which respondents answered on a 5-point scale: every day, 1 to 6 times/wk, 1 to 3 times/month, never, and not applicable (N/A; use air conditioning). These 2009 data were combined with 2005 data to create a 2005–2009 heat stress variable as follows: never heat stress (never or rarely in 2005 and N/A or ≤1–3 times/month in 2009); non-prolonged heat stress (sometimes or often in 2005 and N/A or ≤1–3 times/month in 2009, or vice versa, ie, rarely or never in 2005 and ≥1–6 times/wk in 2009); prolonged heat stress (sometimes or often in 2005 and ≥1–6 times/wk in 2009).

The health outcomes analyzed here were based on self-reports in 2005 and 2009 in response to the question "Have you ever been diagnosed by a doctor as having kidney disease?", with answers of yes and no. We identified incident cases as patients who did not report a diagnosis of kidney disease at baseline in 2005 but did report such a diagnosis in 2009. Also, those who answered yes in 2009 were requested to indicate their age at diagnosis. This enabled an alternative (more restrictive) method to identify incident cases by using reported age at diagnosis and calculated age in 2009 to impute onset of kidney disease after the 2005 baseline. We used the first method of identifying incident cases for our main analyses; the alternative method was used to check our primary results.

The process used to select the cohort members who were analyzed for incidence of kidney disease is shown in Figure 1. The respondents included were those who did not report kidney disease at cohort baseline in 2005, had a paid job in both 2005 and 2009, and answered the questions on heat exposure in 2005 (for analysis of baseline exposure) and both 2005 and 2009 (for analysis of prolonged exposure). They also provided information in 2005 on variables that could confound or modify our estimates of the association between heat stress and kidney disease. These variables were age, sex, education, income, alcohol consumption, smoking, job location, and job type. Because we restricted our study of heat stress to a longitudinal analysis of workers, we did not include individuals who worked in 2005 but did not work in 2009 (Figure 1). In 2009, these 7803 excluded persons reported

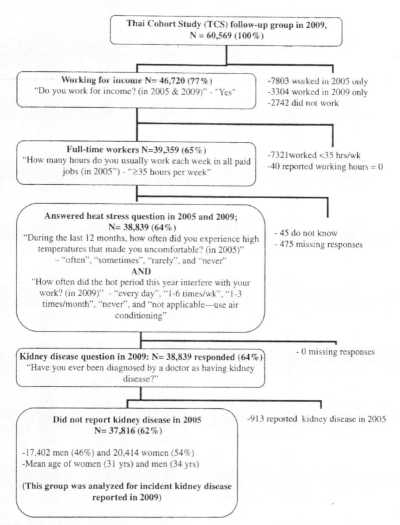

Figure 1. Selection process for analyzed population from the Thai Cohort Study, using data from 2005 and 2009

incident kidney disease at a rate almost identical (1.19%) to that noted in the analyzed cohort of 37 816 persons (1.07%). Thus, there is no evidence that their exclusion lowered our estimate of incident kidney disease.

To prepare for the analysis, we divided heat stress, age, highest education, monthly income, alcohol consumption, smoking, job location, and job type into appropriate categories, and frequencies were tabulated by sex (Table 1). Classification of employment as an office job or physical job was based on the more detailed Thai categories that were reported: skilled and manual workers were coded as physical jobs; all others were coded as office jobs. Body mass index (BMI) was derived from reported height and weight at endpoint (2009) and was classified into 4 categories (underweight, normal weight, overweight, and obese).

Data analysis

Data were digitized using Thai Scandevet software and furth processed using SPSS version 19 and Stata version statistical packages. The initial analysis group included 37 8 cohort members who worked full-time from 2005 throu 2009 and full data sets for heat stress and kidney disea analyses. Subsequent analyses were restricted to 17 402 m who had a significant risk of heat stress and related kidn disease.

Potential explanatory variables were first assessed investigating their association (odds ratios [ORs] and 9 CIs) with the exposure of interest (heat stress in 2005), w results shown graphically for men and women (Figure 2). I this summary analysis, heat stress in 2005 was dichotomiz into often and not often (sometimes/rarely/never). T

Table 1. Reported heat stress at work and socioeconomic, behavioral, and other characteristics in a cohort of 37 816 full-time workers in Thailand

Cohort attributes	Men		Women	
	n	%	n	%
Total	17 402	46.0	20 414	54.0
Heat stress in 2005				
Rarely/Never	7523	43.2	11 288	55.3
Sometimes	5992	34.4	6008	29.4
Often	3887	22.3	3118	15.3
Age group (years)				
15–24	1989	11.4	4411	21.6
25–34	8043	46.2	10 196	50.0
≥35	7370	42.4	5807	28.5
Education				
University	4499	25.9	6472	31.7
Diploma	4422	25.4	6885	33.7
High school	8481	48.7	7057	34.6
Personal income (Baht/month)[a]				
20 001+	2925	16.8	2180	10.7
10 001–20 000	6162	35.4	5573	27.3
7001–10 000	4385	25.2	5450	26.7
<7000	3930	22.6	7211	35.3
Alcohol consumption				
Never	1494	8.6	8033	39.4
Occasional social drinker	12 387	71.2	10 882	53.3
Regular drinker	1971	11.3	124	0.6
Stopped drinking	1550	8.9	1375	6.7
Smoking				
Never smoked	8337	47.9	19 531	95.7
Current smoker	3424	19.7	172	0.8
Ex-smoker	5641	32.4	711	3.5
BMI in 2009				
Normal weight	6966	40.0	11 609	56.9
Underweight	538	3.1	2707	13.3
Overweight	4500	25.9	2844	13.9
Obese	5398	31.0	3254	15.9
Job location				
Bangkok	2576	14.8	3965	19.4
Urban	6712	38.6	7418	36.3
Rural	8114	46.6	9031	44.2
Job type				
Office job	12 393	71.2	16 569	81.2
Physical job	5009	28.8	3845	18.8

US$ 1 = 40 Baht in 2005.

cumulative incidence of kidney disease was then calculated for the period 2005–2009 by age group and sex (Figure 3). Age trends were tested for statistical significance (P-trend 0.05).

For the main analyses, we use logistic regression models with incident kidney disease as the outcome to estimate the association with exposure to heat stress, and calculated crude and adjusted ORs and 95% CIs. Adjusted estimates were derived from models that included all potential explanatory variables. These crude and adjusted models were then subjected to a sensitivity analysis by repeating the estimations using an alternative, more restrictive method of defining incident kidney disease (based on a negative report of kidney disease in 2005, a positive report in 2009, and age at diagnosis of kidney disease reported in 2009, after confirming kidney disease-free status in 2005).

Putative explanatory variables were also evaluated as potential modifiers of heat stress associations by stratified analyses that estimated ORs separately for each variable category. The significant modifiers of heat stress effects on kidney disease were age and job type in men. The final models show the fully adjusted heat stress effect on incidence of kidney disease, stratified by age and job type in male workers.

Ethics

Ethical approval was obtained from Sukhothai Thammathirat Open University Research and Development Institute (protocol 0522/10) and the Australian National University Human Research Ethics Committee (protocol 2004344). Informed, written consent was obtained from all participants.

RESULTS

Characteristics of the cohort

The selection of the analyzed cohort of 2005–2009 workers is presented in Figure 1. Table 1 shows the main characteristics of the 17 402 men (46.0%) and 20 414 women (54.0%) analyzed. The most frequent age range was 25 to 34 years. Women were younger and more likely to work in Bangkok than men (19.4% vs 14.8%). Men were more likely than women to have physical jobs (28.8% vs 18.8%). On average, women had a moderately higher educational level, while men had higher personal incomes. Overall, many more men than women were current smokers (19.7% vs 0.8%) and regular drinkers (11.3% vs 0.6%). More men than women were obese (31.0% vs 15.9%). Exposure to heat stress at baseline (2005) was more common in men than in women (22.3% vs 15.3%). Never experiencing heat stress at work was more frequently reported by women than by men (55.3% vs 43.2%). Further analyses were therefore conducted separately for men and women.

Associations of cohort attributes with heat stress

The associations of cohort attributes with heat stress among men and women in 2005 are presented in Figure 2. The age association with heat stress is shown directly (ie, unadjusted for covariates); other variables tested are mutually adjusted for their association with heat stress. Among both sexes, the prevalence of heat stress exposure varied considerably among subgroups and was notably higher for those with lower incomes and education, regular drinkers, and current smokers. Workers in rural areas more frequently reported heat stress at work than did workers in Bangkok. Those with physical jobs had more heat stress at work than did office workers. For men, all explanatory variables except BMI were significantly associated with heat stress. For women, all explanatory variables except age and education were significantly associated with heat stress. Among workers aged 35 years or older, reporting both heat stress and a physical job was much more common among men (509) than among women (181).

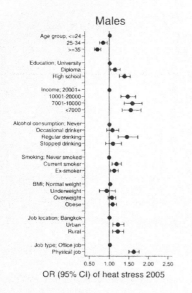
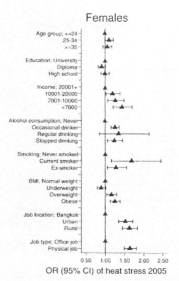

Figure 2. Association of cohort attributes with heat stress in 2005[a]
[a]Odds ratios (ORs) for age not adjusted; other ORs mutually adjusted and adjusted for age

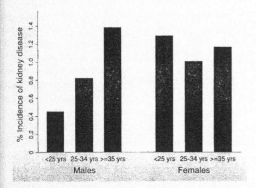

Figure 3. Incidence of kidney disease by age group among male and female workers, 2005–2009

Incidence of kidney disease

The incidence of kidney disease by age group and sex during the 4-year period from 2005 to 2009 is presented in Figure 3. Overall, 405 (1.1%) of the analyzed group developed kidney disease, and the rate was very similar for men and women (1.0% vs 1.1%). Incident kidney disease increased significantly with age for men, reaching 1.4% among those aged 35 years or older (P-trend <0.001); in contrast, there was no age trend for women (P-trend = 0.664). These results show that age is a potential confounder of heat stress effects for men because the proportion of heat stress exposure is greater among younger men, while the incidence of kidney disease increases with age.

Table 2. Associations between heat stress and incid█ kidney disease among men and women work█ full-time

| Heat stress 2005 | Kidney disease | | ORs | | | P-value | 95%█ |
	No.	%	Crude	Age adj.[a]	Adj.[b]		
Men (n = 17 402)	177	1.02					
Never/Rarely	66	0.88	1	1	1		
Sometimes	62	1.03	1.18	1.21	1.19	0.345	0.83–
Often	49	1.26	1.44	1.54*	1.48*	0.045	1.01–
P-trend			0.054	0.025	0.046		
Women (n = 20 414)	228	1.12					
Never/Rarely	130	1.15	1	1	1		
Sometimes	65	1.08	0.94	0.94	0.91	0.548	0.67–
Often	33	1.06	0.92	0.92	0.87	0.471	0.59–
P-trend			0.604	0.606	0.411		

(*P-value <0.05) & (**P-value <0.001).
[a]Associations with heat stress and incidence of kidney disease █ expressed as age-adjusted odds ratios (ORs).
[b]Associations with heat stress and incidence of kidney disease █ expressed as ORs adjusted for explanatory variables: age, alco█ consumption, smoking, body mass index, income, education, job ty█ and job location.

Effect of occupational heat stress on kidney disea█

Table 2 shows crude and adjusted ORs for associati█ between heat stress and incident kidney disease for men █ women. For men, the incidence of kidney disease from 2█ to 2009 was 1.3% among those exposed to heat stress in 20█ compared with 0.9% among those not exposed (adjus█ OR = 1.48, 95% CI 1.01–2.16). For men, there was█ significant dose-response relation between heat stress █ kidney disease (P-trend for adjusted OR = 0.046). There █ no similar trend for women. Therefore, subsequent analyses█

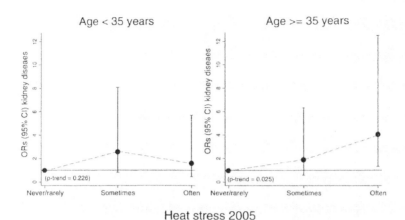

Figure 4. Effect of heat stress in 2005 on incidence of kidney disease in 2009 among men in physical jobs

Table 3. Associations between prolonged heat stress and incident kidney disease among men working full-time

Prolonged heat stress (2005 and 2009)	Men %	Kidney disease		ORs			P-value	95% CI
		No.	%	Crude	Age adj.[a]	Adj.[b]		
Men (n = 17 402)		177	1.02					
Never	31.5	39	0.71	1	1	1		
Non-prolonged heat	42.5	71	0.96	1.35	1.42	1.40	0.099	0.94–2.08
Prolonged heat stress 2005 and 2009	26.0	67	1.48	2.09**	2.25**	2.22**	<0.001	1.48–3.35
P-trend				<0.001	<0.001	<0.001		

*P-value <0.05) & (**P-value <0.001).
Associations with heat stress and incidence of kidney disease are expressed as age-adjusted odds ratios (ORs).
Associations with heat stress and incidence of kidney disease are expressed as ORs adjusted for explanatory variables: age, alcohol consumption, smoking, BMI, income, education, job type and job location.

the effect of heat stress on kidney disease in different age groups and job types were restricted to men.

Compared with men not exposed to heat stress, men with physical jobs who were exposed to heat stress were at higher risk of kidney disease (adjusted OR: 2.57, 95% CI: 1.11–5.93) than were heat-stressed office workers (adjusted OR: 1.26, 95% CI: 0.80–1.98) (data not tabulated). In particular, men aged 35 years or older in physical jobs with frequent heat stress had a particularly high risk of kidney disease (2.6%) compared with the same age group in physical jobs without heat stress (0.7%). In a comparison of these 2 groups, the adjusted OR for kidney disease associated with frequent heat stress was 4.33 (95% CI 1.38–13.60). Moreover, the odds increased with increasing heat stress exposure in this age group (P-trend = 0.025; Figure 4).

Effect of prolonged heat stress on kidney disease

Overall, 26.1% of male workers were exposed to prolonged heat stress in both 2005 and 2009. Working under prolonged heat stress was notably more frequent among those who were younger, had lower incomes and education, regular

drinkers, current smokers, those who worked in rural areas, and particularly those with physical jobs (data not shown); this is the same pattern that was noted above for heat stress at baseline (2005). With increasing exposure to prolonged heat stress among men, the adjusted OR of developing kidney disease also increased (P-trend <0.001). Among those frequently exposed to heat stress, the adjusted OR reached 2.22 (95% CI 1.48–3.35; Table 3). The risk of kidney disease was highest for men aged 35 years or older with frequent prolonged heat stress in physical jobs: 2.2% of such men developed kidney disease compared with 0.4% among those without heat stress (adjusted OR = 5.30, 95% CI 1.17–24.13). In addition, men in this age group with physical jobs had a significantly increased risk of kidney disease with increasing prolonged heat exposure (P-trend = 0.041; Figure 5).

Sensitivity analysis using an alternative method of defining incident kidney disease

The above analyses were repeated using the alternative method of estimating the incidence of kidney disease, ie,

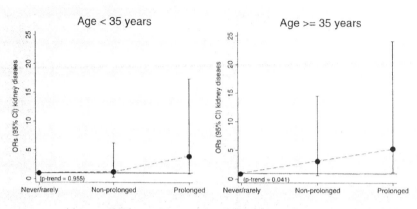

Prolonged heat stress 2005 and 2009

Figure 5. Effect of prolonged heat stress (2005 and 2009) on incidence of kidney disease among men in physical jobs

restricted to those who were negative for kidney disease in 2005, positive in 2009, and, in 2009, reported age at diagnosis (indicating disease onset) after 2005. This method yielded 30% fewer cases of incident kidney disease among full-time workers (283 vs 405), which reduced statistical power. Crude and adjusted ORs for incident kidney disease associated with heat stress in 2005 among men and women were almost identical to corresponding ORs reported in Table 2, ie, using the primary method of estimating incidence. In addition, using the 2005–2009 heat stress variable, the effect of prolonged heat stress among men was identical to the corresponding OR in Table 3 (adjusted OR: 2.22), and the overall effects of heat stress (never vs non-prolonged vs prolonged) remained highly significant for trend (<0.001).

DISCUSSION

Several findings in the present study of occupational heat stress and kidney disease were notable. Many Thai workers (18%) in the cohort reported exposure to heat stress at baseline in 2005, and such exposure was more common in men than in women. Furthermore, there was an association between reported heat stress and 4-year (2005–2009) incidence of kidney disease in men but not in women. This important finding was validated by showing almost identical results when defining incidence using an alternative method based on reported age at diagnosis. These results were tested yet again by including only kidney disease cases with an institution named for diagnosis, and again the results were similar (data not shown). We also found that the risk of kidney disease increased with increasing dose of prolonged heat stress exposure in men and that the risk was higher among those aged 35 years or older and those with physical jobs. Older men in physical jobs had a 5.3-times increase in the risk of incident kidney disease.

Overall, these epidemiologic results remained substan[tial] and statistically significant when adjusted for a vari[ety] of potential explanatory variables (age, income, educati[on], alcohol consumption, smoking, BMI, job type, and location). These included adjustments for socioecono[mic] status—which has been shown in other studies to [be] an important correlate of kidney disease[21,22]—and smoking.[23]

The main advantage of this study is its access to a la[rge] nationwide cohort of 17 402 male and 20 414 female full-t[ime] workers in Thailand. It reasonably accurately represents m[ale] and female Thais of working age with regard to geograp[hic] location, age, and socioeconomic status.[18–20] Cohort mem[bers] are better educated than average Thais of the same age [and] sex, which enabled us to gather complex heat exposure [and] health outcome data by questionnaire. The cohort showe[d a] wide range of values for the variables of interest, wh[ich] allowed us to investigate the relationship between heat st[ress] at work and health outcomes. Furthermore, the follow[-up] study allows us to analyze incidence data and to catego[rize] heat exposure by degree of prolongation.

Another strength of this study is that self-report[ed] heat stress were unlikely to be biased, as the questionna[ire] included a substantial number of questions on diffe[rent] exposures and diseases, and thus respondents would [be] unaware of any connection to kidney disease. Also, [they] would not benefit by over- or under-reporting.

We found an association of reported heat stress at w[ork] and reported kidney disease in tropical Thailand. Howe[ver,] this important overall finding has some limitations. Our s[tudy] could not directly establish that kidney disease resulted [from] heat stress. However, the longitudinal data allow us to be [sure] that heat stress exposure preceded kidney disease outco[me.] Unfortunately, the source and nature of heat stress, and ac[tual] work conditions, were not characterized in detail. We [were] not able to directly measure, or further investigate, work environments or kidney disease outcomes and hence this report must be regarded as preliminary. Therefore, there is a need for more detailed observations in informative, heat-stressed work settings and for studies of actual kidney disease to validate our findings, explore underlying mechanisms, and further characterize associated kidney disease.

As noted above, we need to collect more detailed health and environmental information from various work settings in Thailand. We should begin with an informative sample of the cohort analyzed in this report. The sample should include both sexes, a variety of occupations, and participants aged 35 years or older in urban and rural settings of major regions of Thailand. The sample must also include persons with or without heat stress and with or without kidney disease. We could collect detailed information on heat stress, water intake and dehydration, and reported kidney disease. Wet-bulb temperature measurements at workplaces of a subsample of affected individuals would permit us to document heat stress, and medical records could document kidney disease and its characteristics. Such a study should lead to more detailed assessment of other (non-cohort) samples of at-risk heat-stressed workers and would include extensive clinical examinations of the kidney to conclusively document renal effects.

Our findings complement those of other reports that highlight the growing importance of kidney disease in Thailand. The Thai Ministry of Public Health reports a 70% increase in hospitalizations for kidney disease (acute renal failure, chronic renal failure, and kidney stone) from 2005 (180 779 cases) to 2009 (305 130 cases).[24] The Fourth National Health Examination Survey Report 2008–2009 found that the prevalence of renal failure was 1.2% among Thai adults, and the rates were similar for men and women.[25] In our cohort, the incidence of reported doctor-diagnosed kidney disease was 1.1%, with similar rates for men and women. However, kidney disease among women did not appear to involve heat stress and was probably related to female anatomy—short urethras increase the incidence of urinary tract infection. However, among men, occupational heat stress was a risk factor for kidney disease. This may be because, compared with women, the proportions of men who work in physical jobs and work outdoors are higher.[26] Women have more body fat and are consequently more sensitive to heat. Men could also be less aware of dehydration and engage more-intense muscular activity, resulting in hyperuricemia and rhabdomyolysis, both of which pose a threat to kidney health.[27] It should also be noted that men appear to be more susceptible to heat stress, as shown by data from a 2003 heat wave in France.[28]

Although there is a high prevalence of kidney disease among outdoor workers in the tropics, occupational heat stress-related kidney disease has received little attention.[29] In an Italian study, Borghi et al[30] showed that chronic

dehydration among glass-industry workers exposed to heat stress was a risk factor for kidney stones. In a Brazilian study, Atan et al[31] found that male steel-industry workers in high-temperature areas had a 9-fold risk of kidney stones compared with those working at room temperature. A study by Gracia-Trabanino et al[32] found a high prevalence of chronic kidney disease among coastal male farmers in Central American countries. Recently, other reports have shown an association between extreme temperature (heat waves) and kidney disease in a temperate city.[4,33] In addition, there are reports that high ambient temperature is associated with kidney stone occurrence in some populations.[26,34,35]

Our finding of an association between occupational heat stress and kidney disease is new for Thailand. However, the potential links of high occupational heat exposure to health effects in Thailand was recently discussed in an article by Langkulsen et al.[17] The heat stress effects detected in our study translate to a significant public health burden of preventable heat-related kidney disease among Thai workers. This is particularly important at present because we expect that the existing problem will worsen if global warming continues and that workplaces will become even more thermally stressful. More attention is needed to the health of tropical workers, especially older male workers doing physical jobs during hot weather or under prolonged heat stress. Maintaining hydration must be emphasized for physical workers in Thailand, and this requires a health-behavior intervention. In addition, construction of buildings for workplaces must account for indoor climate while minimizing the use of energy-consuming air conditioning systems.

In our longitudinal analysis of Thai Cohort Study data, we conclude there is an association between exposure to occupational heat stress and kidney disease among men. The underlying mechanisms require further study. A rapid increase is kidney disease is already occurring in tropical Thailand. Heat stress should be regarded as a potential cause, and global warming will increase the risk.

ACKNOWLEDGMENTS

This study was supported by the International Collaborative Research Grants Scheme, with joint grants from the Wellcome Trust UK (GR071587MA) and the Australian NHMRC (268055), and by a global health grant from the NHMRC (585426). We thank the staff at Sukhothai Thammathirat Open University (STOU), who assisted with student contact, and the STOU students who are participating in the cohort study. We also thank Dr Bandit Thinkamrop and his team from Khon Kaen University for guiding us through the complex data processing. Finally, we thank Prof Carl-Gustaf Elinder and Dr Keith Dear for their helpful comments.

Conflicts of interest: None declared.

REFERENCES

1. Kjellstrom T, Butler AJ, Lucas RM, Bonita R. Public health impact of global heating due to climate change: potential effects on chronic non-communicable diseases. Int J Public Health. 2010;55:97–103.

2. Hansen AL, Bi P, Ryan P, Nitschke M, Pisaniello D, Tucker G. The effect of heat waves on hospital admissions for renal disease in a temperate city of Australia. Int J Epidemiol. 2008; 37(6):1359–65.

3. Basu R. High ambient temperature and mortality: A review of epidemiologic studies from 2001 to 2008. Environ Health. 2009;8:40.

4. Knowlton K, Rotkin-Ellman M, King G, Margolis HG, Smith D, Solomon G, et al. The 2006 California heat wave: impacts on hospitalizations and emergency department visits. Environ Health Perspect. 2009;117(1):61–7.

5. Tawatsupa B, Lim LL, Kjellstrom T, Seubsman SA, Sleigh A; The Thai Cohort Study Team. The association between overall health, psychological distress, and occupational heat stress among a large national cohort of 40,913 Thai workers. Glob Health Action. 2010;3:5034.

6. Parsons K. Human thermal environments: the effects of hot, moderate, and cold environments on human health, comfort and performance. 2nd ed. New York: CRC Press; 2003.

7. Schrier RW, Hano J, Keller HI, Finkel RM, Gilliland PF, Cirksena WJ, et al. Renal, metabolic, and circulatory responses to heat and exercise. Ann Intern Med. 1970;73(2):213–23.

8. Brikowski TH, Lotan Y, Pearle MS. Climate-related increase in the prevalence of urolithiasis in the United States. Proc Natl Acad Sci USA. 2008;105(28):9841–6.

9. Semenza JC. Acute renal failure during heat waves. Am J Prev Med. 1999;17(1):97.

10. Semenza JC, McCullough JE, Flanders WD, McGeehin MA, Lumpkin JR. Excess hospital admissions during the July 1995 heat wave in Chicago. Am J Prev Med. 1999;16(4):269–77.

11. Al-Tawheed AR, Al-Awadi KA, Kehinde EO, Abdul-Halim H, Al-Hunayan A, Ali Y, et al. Anuria secondary to hot weather-induced hyperuricaemia: diagnosis and management. Ann Saudi Med. 2003;23(5):283–7.

12. Public Health Statistic [database on the Internet]. Bureau of Policy and Strategy, Ministry of Public Health, Thailand. 2007 [updated 2010 May 5; cited 2011 April 25]. Available from: http://bps.ops.moph.go.th/Healthinformation/statistic50/statistic50.html (in Thai).

13. Tanthanuch M, Apiwatgaroon A, Pripatnanont C. Urinary tract calculi in southern Thailand. J Med Assoc Thai. 2005;88(1): 80–5.

14. Sriboonlue P, Prasongwatana V, Chata K, Tungsanga K. Prevalence of upper urinary tract stone disease in a rural community of north-eastern Thailand. Br J Urol. 1992;69(3): 240–4.

15. Limsakul A, Goes JI. Empirical evidence for interannual and longer period variability in Thailand surface air temperatures. Atmos Res. 2008;87(2):89–102.

16. Kjellstrom T, Holmer I, Lemke B. Workplace heat stress, health and productivity—an increasing challenge for low and middle-income countries during climate change. Glob Health Acti 2009;2.

17. Langkulsen U, Vichit-Vadakan N, Taptagaporn S. Health imp of climate change on occupational health and productivity Thailand. Glob Health Action. 2010;3:5607.

18. Sleigh AC, Seubsman SA, Bain C; Thai Cohort Study Tea Cohort profile: the Thai cohort of 87,134 open univers students. Int J Epidemiol. 2008;37:266–72.

19. Seubsman S, Yiengprugsawan V, Sleigh A; The Thai Coh Study Team. A large national Thai Cohort Study of Health-Risk Transition based on Sukhothai Thammath Open University students. ASEAN Journal of Open Distai Learning. 2011; (in press).

20. Seubsman SA, Kelly M, Sleigh A, Peungson J, Chokkanapital Vilainerun D, et al. Methods used for successful follow-up i large scale national cohort study in Thailand. BMC Res No 2011;4:166.

21. Fored CM, Ejerblad E, Fryzek JP, Lambe M, Lindblad P, Ny O, et al. Socio economic status and chronic renal failure population-based case-control study in Sweden. Nephrol I Transplant. 2003;18(1):82–8.

22. White SL, McGeechan K, Jones M, Cass A, Chadban Polkinghorne KR, et al. Socioeconomic disadvantage and kid disease in the United States, Australia, and Thailand. Ar Public Health. 2008;98(7):1306–13.

23. Orth SR, Ogata H, Ritz E. Smoking and the kidney. Neph Dial Transplant. 2000;15(10):1509–11.

24. Number and Rates of in-patients according to 21 groups causes from Health Service Units, Ministry of Public Health 1,000 Population, 2005 and 2009 [database on the Interr Bureau of Policy and Strategy, Ministry of Public Hea Thailand. 2009. Available from: http://bps.ops.moph.go Healthinformation (in Thai).

25. Aekpalakorn W, Porapakkham Y, Taneepanichskul S, Pakjar H, Satheannoppakao W, Thaikla K. The Fourth National He Examination Survey, 2008–9. Nonthaburi, Thailand: He System Research Institute; 2011 (in Thai).

26. Fakheri RJ, Goldfarb DS. Ambient temperature as a contrib to kidney stone formation: Implications of global warm Kidney Int. 2011;79(11):1178–85.

27. Uberoi HS, Dugal JS, Kasthuri AS, Kolhe VS, Kumar AK, C SA. Acute renal failure in severe exertional rhabdomyoly J Assoc Physicians India. 1991;39(9):677–9.

28. Hémon D, Jougla E. Excess mortality related to the heatwav August 2003, Progress Report, Estimation of mortality major epidemiological characteristics. Paris, France: Ins National de la Santé et de la Recherche Médicale (INSER 2003 (in France).

29. Pin NT, Ling NY, Siang LH. Dehydration from outdoor w and urinary stones in a tropical environment. Occup Med (Lo 1992;42(1):30–2.

30. Borghi L, Meschi T, Amato F, Novarini A, Romanelli A, Cig F. Hot occupation and nephrolithiasis. J Urol. 1993;15C 1757–60.

31. Atan L, Andreoni C, Ortiz V, Silva EK, Pitta R, Atan F, e High kidney stone risk in men working in steel industry at temperatures. Urology. 2005;65(5):858–61.

32. Gracia-Trabanino R, Domínguez J, Jansà JM, Oliver

Proteinuria and chronic renal failure in the coast of El Salvador: detection with low cost methods and associated factors. Nefrologia. 2005;25:31–8.

33. Hansen A, Bi P, Nitschke M, Ryan P, Pisaniello D, Tucker G. The effect of heatwaves on ambulance callouts in Adelaide, South Australia. Epidemiology. 2011;22(1):S14–5.

34. Cervellin G, Comelli I, Comelli D, Cortellini P, Lippi G, Meschi T, et al. Regional short-term climate variations influence on the number of visits for renal colic in a large urban Emergency Department: Results of a 7-year survey. Intern Emerg Med. 2011;6(2):141–7.

35. Garcia-Pina R, Tobías Garcés A, Sanz Navarro J, Navarro Sánchez C, Garcia-Fulgueiras A. Effect of weather temperature on hospital emergencies in the Region of Murcia, Spain, throughout the 2000–2005 and its use in epidemiological surveillance. Rev Esp Salud Publica. 2008;82(2):153–66 (in Spanish).

CHAPTER 6: HEAT STRESS AND WELL-BEING[4]

Increasing heat stress is an important issue of public health concern. The effects of daily heat stress exposure can have a major influence on human daily activities but there is limited information regarding the impact on overall health and well-being. This study is based on 2009 data from an ongoing national Thai Cohort Study that began in 2005. This chapter aims to examine the association between hot season heat stress interference with daily activities (sleeping, work, travel, housework, exercise) and three graded holistic health outcomes (energy, emotions, life satisfaction). This chapter shows that the tropical Thailand has substantial heat stress impacts on health and wellbeing. Increasing temperatures from climate change as well as the growing urban population could significantly worsen the situation in this country.

[4] A version of Chapter 6 has been published. Tawatsupa B, Yiengprugsawan V, Kjellstrom T, Seubsman S-a, Sleigh A, the Thai Cohort Study Team (2012) Heat stress, health, and wellbeing: findings from a large national cohort of Thai adults. *BMJ Open* 2:e001396. DOI: 10.1136/bmjopen-2012-001396.

Heat stress, health and well-being: findings from a large national cohort of Thai adults

Benjawan Tawatsupa,[1,2] Vasoontara Yiengprugsawan,[1] Tord Kjellstrom,[1,3] Sam-ang Seubsman,[4] Adrian Sleigh,[1] the Thai Cohort Study Team

te: Tawatsupa B,
prugsawan V,
strom T, et al. Heat
s, health and well-being:
gs from a large national
rt of Thai adults. BMJ
2012;2:e001396.
0.1136/bmjopen-2012-
96

epublication history and
onal material for this
are available online.
w these files please
he journal online
/dx.doi.org/10.1136/
pen-2012-001396).

ved 30 April 2012
ted 5 October 2012

mbered affiliations see
article

pondence to
van Tawatsupa;
708@hotmail.com

ABSTRACT

Objectives: This study aims to examine the association between self-reported heat stress interference with daily activities (sleeping, work, travel, housework and exercise) and three graded-holistic health and well-being outcomes (energy, emotions and life satisfaction).

Design: A cross-sectional study.

Setting: The setting is tropical and developing countries as Thailand, where high temperature and high humidity are common, particularly during the hottest seasons.

Participants: This study is based on an ongoing national Thai Cohort Study of distance-learning open-university adult students (N=60 569) established in 2005 to study the health-risk transition.

Primary and secondary outcome measures: Health impacts from heat stress in our study are categorised as physical health impacts (energy levels), mental health impacts (emotions) and well-being (life satisfaction). For each health and well-being outcome we report ORs and 95% CIs using multinomial logistic regression adjusting for a wide array of potential confounders.

Results: Negative health and well-being outcomes (low-energy level, emotional problems and low life satisfaction) associated with increasing frequency of heat stress interfering with daily activities. Adjusted ORs for emotional problems were between 1.5 and 4.8 and in general worse than energy level (between 1.31 and 2.91) and life satisfaction (between 1.10 and 2.49). The worst health outcomes were when heat interfered with sleeping, followed by interference with daily travel, work, housework and exercise.

Conclusions: In tropical Thailand there already are substantial heat stress impacts on health and well-being. Increasing temperatures from climate change plus the ageing and urbanisation of the population could significantly worsen the situation. There is a need to improve public health surveillance and public awareness regarding the risks of heat stress in daily life.

ARTICLE SUMMARY

Article focus
- To examine the association between self-reported heat stress interference with daily activities (sleeping, work, travel, housework and exercise) during hot season and three graded holistic health outcomes (energy, emotions and life satisfaction) in Thailand.

Key messages
- Negative health and well-being outcomes (low energy level, emotional problems and low life satisfaction) associated with increasing frequency of heat stress interfering with daily activities.
- The worst health outcomes were when heat interfered with sleeping, followed by interference with daily travel, work, housework and exercise.
- The results from this study point to the need for improving public health surveillance and public awareness regarding the risks of heat stress in daily life in a tropical country like Thailand.

Strengths and limitations of this study
- The possible limitation of self-reports, but note that questions on heat stress and health outcomes were in different parts of the questionnaire.
- The strength of this study is its large scale with participation from a national group of adults embedded in the socioeconomic mainstream of Thai society and used the comprehensive questionnaire which captures a detailed assessment of health and an array of geodemographic, environmental and social attributes.

Increasing heat stress has substantial adverse effects on population mortality and morbidity.[2–5] This information is from developed and temperate countries[3] and leaves unanswered questions for tropical and developing countries where high temperature and humidity are common. Furthermore, heat stress in tropical cities is increasing due to urban heat island effects caused by industrial development and urbanisation in developing countries.[6]

Heat stress can have a major influence on daily human activities. The body absorbs

INTRODUCTION

Over the last decade interest has grown in the impact of global warming on human health.[1]

external heat due to high air temperature and humidity, low air movement and high solar radiation; as well, some physical activities generate heat internally.[7] Excess heat exposure during normal daily activities creates a high risk of recurrent dehydration and can cause other effects on physical health (eg, exhaustion, heat cramps, heat stroke or death).[7] Heat stress affects mood, increases psychological distress and mental health problems,[8-10] and also reduces key human psychological performance variables.[11]

Other heat stress impacts may arise from increased mistakes in daily activities and accidental injuries. As well, disturbed sleep and degraded physical performance from heat exhaustion reduce work capacity and lead to loss of income.[8 12 13] Populations at risk of heat stress are not only the elderly but also young people and adults who are more likely to carry out heavy labour outdoors or work indoors without air conditioning or other effective cooling systems during the hot season.[8 12 14]

In tropical Thailand, hot and humid conditions are common, especially in the hot season (March–June). The monthly maximum, mean and minimum temperatures averaged from 1999 to 2008 were around 33°C, 27°C and 22°C, respectively, with the averaged relative humidity at 75%. The monthly maximum temperatures averaged during 10 years varied little by region (32–33°C) and were highest in the North region during April (40°C) and lowest in the same region during December (24°C).[15]

Global warming (or 'global heating' may be a better description in relation to Thailand) is now causing increasing alarm in many tropical areas. For example, from 1951 to 2003, the monthly mean maximum temperature in Thailand increased by 0.56°C and the monthly mean minimum temperature increased even more at 1.44°C.[16] Heat stress is already a concern in Thailand and the observed trends indicate further increase in air temperature.[17] A recent study of occupational heat stress in Thailand by Langkulsen et al[18] revealed a very serious problem ('extreme caution' or 'danger') in an array of work settings (they tested a pottery factory, a power plant, a knife manufacture site, a construction site and an agricultural site).

Heat stress in Thailand, its effects and pathways to exposure have been reported for two cities [19 20] and for workers.[10 21] However, there is no available information on how much heat interferes with normal daily activities and heat stress effects on health and well-being in the general Thai population. Here we report an investigation of association between heat stress interference with daily activities and health and well-being in a large national cohort of young and middle-aged Thai adults.

METHODS
Study population
In 2005, a baseline questionnaire was mailed out to adult students enrolled at Sukhothai Thammathirat Open University. The questionnaire was developed by a multidisciplinary team in both Thailand and Austr[...] cover a wide range of topics for a longitudinal st[...] the Thai Health-Risk Transition—transformati[...] the health-risk and outcome pattern in Thaila[...] infectious diseases recede and chronic diseases e[...] Overall, 87 134 distance-learning students [...] 15–87 years responded from all areas of Thailand. [...] participants were generally similar to the popula[...] Thailand, especially in the 30–39 years age group, [...] ratio, income and geographical location.[22]

Data collected included demographic, socioeco[...] and geographic characteristics, physical and [...] health status, personal well-being, health-service u[...] behaviours, injuries, diet, physical activity and [...] background. A 4-year follow-up was conducted i[...] and the next one is due in 2013.

This report is based on the 2009 follow-up [...] included questions on heat interference with [...] daily activities. The heat stress and health outcom[...] sures (both described below) were in different p[...] the questionnaire. They could not easily be linke[...] respondent's mind so answers on these issues wer[...] pendent. Covariates analysed are described wi[...] results and include age, sex, marital status, geog[...] location, work status, smoking, drinking and bod[...] index.

Measures of heat stress
Questions related to heat stress were as follows[...] often did the hot period this year interfere with t[...] lowing activities?' (1) sleeping; (2) housework; (3[...] travel; (4) work and (5) exercise. Responses we[...] applicable—use air conditioning', 'never', '1–3[...] per month', '1–6 times per week' and 'every day'. [...] study, heat interference means heat stress caus[...] uncomfortable feeling when doing those daily ac[...] For analysis, we grouped self-reported heat stre[...] 'never', 'sometimes' (1–3 times per month), and [...] (1–6 times per week or every day).

Measures of health and well-being outcomes
Health is defined by WHO as 'a complete state o[...] ical, mental and social well-being and not mere[...] absence of disease or infirmity'.[23] Health impact [...] heat stress in our study are categorised as physical [...] impacts (eg, energy levels), mental health impac[...] emotions) and well-being (eg, life satisfaction). [...] three outcomes were selected because they mat[...] holistic WHO health definition and represent [...] mental health states. Many other more specific d[...] would be expected to follow adverse outcomes fo[...] health measures (see Discussion section).

To measure the physical and mental health i[...] we used two questions from the standard M[...] Outcomes Short Form Instrument (SF8) as f[...] *Energy*: 'During the past four weeks, how much [...] did you have?' Responses were 'very much', 'quite [...] 'some', 'a little' and 'none'. For analysis we con[...]

last two categories. *Emotions:* 'During the past four ·ks, how much have you been bothered by emotional ·blems (such as feeling anxious, depressed, or irrit-
·)?' Responses were 'not at all', 'slightly', 'moder-
·y', 'quite a lot' and 'extremely'. For analysis the last
categories were combined. To measure *Well-being* we
·d a standardised question:[24][25] 'Thinking about your
· life and personal circumstances, how satisfied are
·with your life as a whole?' Scores range from 0
·mpletely dissatisfied') to 10 ('completely satisfied').

· processing and statistical analysis

·a scanning and editing involved checking the actual
·stionnaire response against its digital value using
· Scandevet, SQL and SPSS software. For analysis we
·d multinomial logistic regression reporting ORs
·usted for potential confounders) based on Stata
·[26] For all three fundamental health outcomes
·rgy, emotions and well-being), the multinomial
·ession estimates the odds with which each of three
·easingly severe abnormalities occurs relative to the
·s of an optimal outcome. Individuals with missing
·were excluded and so the totals presented vary a
·according to the information available.

al considerations

·cs approval was obtained from Sukhothai
·nmathirat Open University Research and
·lopment Institute (protocol 0522/10) and the
·ralian National University Human Research Ethics
·mittee (protocol 2009/570). Informed written
·ent was obtained from all participants.

·LTS

·irst compared the 2005–2009 cohort to those who
·ped out in 2009 (data not shown). The two groups
·similar for age, sex ratio, employment, income and
·h outcomes studied here (energy levels, emotional
·lems and life satisfaction). Sociodemographic and
·h characteristics of the 60 569 cohort members fol-
·d up in 2009 are presented in table 1. There were
·ly more women (54.8%), 70% were aged less than
·ars and 55.3% were married. Nearly 20% reported
·ehold monthly income of less than 10 000 Baht
·$US) per month, 73.2% reported doing paid
·and 56% resided in urban areas. Health-risk
·viours—regular smoking or regular alcohol
·ing—were reported by 7.7% and 13.7%, respect-
·By Asian standards,[27] half the cohort members
·in the normal weight range, 9.5% were under-
·t, 18.8% were overweight and 22.1% were obese.
·noted that prevalence of 'often' heat interference
·ch daily activity are not much different in different
·ns of Thailand (33–42% for daily travel, 29–38%
·ork, 26–32% for housework, 23–29% for sleeping
·2–28% for exercise). Daily activities and heat inter-
·ce frequency categories are summarised in table 2.

Table 1 Sociodemographic and health characteristics of Thai cohort members in 2009

Cohort characteristics	N=60569	Per cent
Demographic characteristics		
Sex	Male	45.3
	Female	54.8
Age (year)	≤29	27.4
	30–39	42.6
	40+	30.0
Marital status	Married	55.3
	Never married	37.9
	Separated, divorced and widowed	6.8
Sociogeographic characteristics		
Monthly income (Baht)*	≤10000	18.8
	10001–20000	22.4
	20001–30000	35.7
	>30000	23.1
Work status	Doing paid work	73.2
	Unpaid family workers	7.3
	Seeking work	2.2
	Others	17.3
Residence	Rural residence	44.0
	Urban residence	56.0
Health-risk behaviours		
	Regular smokers	7.7
	Regular alcohol drinkers	13.7
Body mass index (kg/m²)		
	Underweight (<18.5)	9.5
	Normal (18.5–22.9)	49.5
	Overweight at risk (23–24.9)	18.8
	Obese (25+)	22.1

*Household monthly income in 2009 (US$=35 Baht).

Heat interference 'often' was reported (in order of frequency) by 37.5% for daily travel, 34.5% for work,
29.9% for housework, 27.4% for sleeping and 25.9% for
exercise. Health and well-being frequency outcomes are
reported in table 3: 37.6% reported being very satisfied

Table 2 Daily activities and heat interference category among Thai cohort members in 2009

Daily activities N=60569	Heat interference (%)			
	Not applicable*	Never	Sometimes	Often
Sleeping	15.7	24.3	32.5	27.4
Housework	1.3	37.1	31.7	29.9
Daily travel	3.0	33.7	25.8	37.5
Work	14.0	30.3	21.2	34.5
Exercise	0.8	43.1	30.1	25.9

*Use air conditioner.

Table 3 Health and well-being outcomes among Thai cohort members in 2009

Outcomes N=60569	Per cent
Overall life satisfaction (score ranged from 0 to 10)	
9–10 very satisfied (highest)	37.6
8 (high)	28.8
6–7 (medium)	21.7
0–5 not very satisfied (low)	12.0
Energy level in the past 4 weeks	
Very much	14.9
Quite a lot	44.0
Some	32.0
A little or none	9.1
Emotional problems in the past 4 weeks	
Not at all	11.3
Slightly	48.4
Moderately	25.8
Quite a lot/extremely	14.5

with their life, around 15% reported having very much energy in the past 4 weeks and close to 11% reported no emotional problems in the past 4 weeks.

Daily activities show a clear trend connecting increasing heat interference with worse health and well-being (table 4). For example, cohort members who experienced heat interference 'often' while sleeping reported 'extreme' emotional problems (38.9%) much more frequently than 'no' emotional problems (16.4%). A similar pattern for 'little or none' energy levels was found for those reporting heat interference 'often' while sleeping (36.1% vs 22%) and the same trend was observed for life satisfaction (39.8% vs 22.2%). Daily travel and work have also shown strong gradients connecting frequent heat interference and worse health outcomes.

The multinomial logistic regression, adjusting for a wide array of potential confounders (see footnote in table 5), supported the descriptive results. For all three health outcomes, when each of the three graded-adverse outcome categories is compared with the optimal outcome, the relative odds ranged from 1.10 to 4.81. Furthermore, most ORs show a dose–response (for each health outcome, more heat interference associates more strongly with a given grade of abnormality). And 95% CIs for all ORs indicated statistical significance. So heat stress interfering with normal daily activities (sleep, housework, travel, work and exercise) associates with adverse outcomes for all three holistic measures of health. For example, reporting heat interference 'often' while sleeping was strongly associated with 'little or none' energy (OR=2.23, 95% CI 2.02 to 2.46), 'extreme' emotional problems (OR=4.81, 95% CI 4.32 to 5.36) and 'low' life satisfaction (OR=2.49, 95% CI 2.28 to 2.71). At work, reporting heat interference 'often' was associated with 'little or none' energy (OR=2.45, 95% CI

2.22 to 2.71) and 'extreme' emotional problems (OR=3.64, 95% CI 3.31 to 4.00). Similar results found during daily travel and doing housework. A tically significant association was also found for inference during exercise but the magnitude of effect was lower than for other activities.

DISCUSSION

Our study shows that climate-related heat stress in ical Thailand associated with self-reported health well-being if the heat interfered with daily activities as sleep, housework, travel, work and exercise. The study group included young and middle-age Thai a mostly doing paid work, with a little over half resid urban areas. These cohort members are active and 20% report often experiencing heat interferenc daily activities during the hot season. Daily trave work were sources of heat stress more often than activities, probably because they involve time spe traffic or outdoors during hot periods. Other act such as housework have less heat stress than daily and work, perhaps because these activities are based where air-conditioning or other ventilati available.

We found those who report higher levels of heat interference with daily activities tend to also be the who have adverse health and well-being outcome life satisfaction, low energy level and worse emo problems). ORs of heat stress effects across all daily ities for emotional problems are between 1.55 and and in general are worse than energy level of (between 1.31 and 2.91) and life satisfaction of (between 1.10 and 2.49). The worst health out were for heat stress while sleeping followed by heat for daily travel, work, housework and exercise.

Our data are based on self-report by educated and we note that questions on heat stress and outcomes were in different parts of the question Findings show strong and highly consistent trends cially for adverse health effects of frequent heat in ence during sleep, daily travel and work. Else we have completed detailed analyses of associ between heat stress and self-reported health outc in the cohort using the questions from SF8.[16] studied outcomes in this report were holistic funda tal measures of health. We can expect that those had abnormal findings would also (already or e ally) manifest other more specific chronic diseases as depression, obesity, hypertension and kidney di If so, the eventual burden of heat-related disease w higher than currently recognised.[28–30]

Our findings add to some previous report working in hot environments which found that stress significantly reduced people's motivation their work. Lan et al[31] assessed office workers' pe tions of thermal environment, emotions, well-bein motivation to work, and found that participants

Tawatsupa B, Yiengprugsawan V, Kjellstrom T, et al. BMJ Open 2012;2:e001396. doi:10.1136/bmjopen-2012-

Table 4   Frequency of heat interference with daily activities by health and well-being outcomes among cohort members

Daily activities and heat interference category	Health and well-being outcomes N=60569											
	Percentage of life satisfaction score ranged from 0 to 10				Percentage of energy level in the past 4 weeks				Percentage of emotional problems in the past 4 weeks			
	9–10 Highest	8 High	6–7 Medium	0–5 Low	Very much	Quite a lot	Some	Little/none	Not at all	Slightly	Moderate	Extreme
Sleep (n)	(22132)	(17024)	(12770)	(7052)	(8833)	(26142)	(18968)	(5378)	(6684)	(28752)	(15297)	(8603)
Never	29.5	22.9	19.7	19.7	33.2	25.3	20.2	19.6	38.6	25.4	19.3	18.6
Sometimes	30.2	34.7	35	30.1	29.9	34	32.5	29.4	25.5	34.3	33.9	29.3
Often	22.2	25.7	32.2	39.8	22	24.5	31.5	36.1	16.4	24	32.3	38.9
Housework (n)	(22094)	(16992)	(12748)	(7029)	(8827)	(26085)	(18924)	(5364)	(6668)	(28683)	(15273)	(8590)
Never	43.6	36.2	31	30.4	46.6	39.1	31.9	30.7	53.2	38.9	31.1	29.7
Sometimes	28	34.4	35.4	30.2	26.1	32.6	33.3	31	24.2	32.8	33.6	30.4
Often	27	28.2	32.5	38.4	25.9	27.1	33.6	36.8	20.8	27.1	33.9	38.9
Daily travel (n)	(22111)	(16994)	(12739)	(7018)	(8829)	(26082)	(18931)	(5355)	(6668)	(28692)	(15275)	(8576)
Never	40.1	33.2	27.5	26.1	42.7	35.6	28.3	28	49.7	35.7	27.8	25.2
Sometimes	24.4	27.6	27.4	23.3	23.1	27.1	26	23.1	21.6	27.3	16.7	22.4
Often	32.4	35.8	42.6	48.7	31.4	34.1	42.6	46.1	24.7	34	42.7	50
Work (n)	(22100)	(17000)	(12744)	(7018)	(8831)	(26101)	(18923)	(5362)	(6668)	(28706)	(15279)	(8579)
Never	36.4	29.6	24.4	23.9	38.9	32	25.7	24.2	45.5	32.1	24.6	22.6
Sometimes	20.3	21.8	22.8	19.2	19.1	22.5	21	19.1	17.1	22.5	22	18.9
Often	29.8	33.2	38.5	44.9	30	31.4	38.7	41.5	23.7	31.1	39.7	44.7
Exercise (n)	(22080)	(16966)	(12724)	(7016)	(8825)	(26065)	(18895)	(5333)	(6664)	(28668)	(15239)	(8561)
Never	46.8	42.6	38.8	41	49.8	43.5	39.7	42.8	55.2	43.9	38.1	40.2
Sometimes	27.8	31.8	33	28.2	24.9	31.1	31.7	28.5	23.7	30.8	32.4	28.9
Often	24.6	24.8	27.4	30.2	24.7	24.6	27.7	27.9	20.1	24.5	28.8	30.2

Table 5 Association between heat interference with daily activities and health and well-being outcomes among cohort members

	Adjusted* OR and 95% CI								
	Life satisfaction (score 0–10)†			Energy level in the past 4 weeks			Emotional problems in the past 4 weeks		
Heat interference category N=60569	High versus highest	Medium versus highest	Low versus highest	Quite a lot versus very much	Some versus very much	Little/none versus very much	Slightly versus not at all	Moderate versus not at all	Extreme versus not at all
Sleep									
Never	Ref	Ref	Ref	Ref	Ref	Ref	Ref	Ref	Ref
Sometimes	1.46	1.66	1.42	1.48	1.76	1.65	1.94	2.48	2.23
	(1.37 to 1.55)	(1.55 to 1.78)	(1.30 to 1.55)	(1.38 to 1.59)	(1.63 to 1.90)	(1.48 to 1.84)	(1.80 to 2.10)	(2.28 to 2.70)	(2.02 to 2.46)
Often	1.50	2.10	2.49	1.52	2.44	2.91	2.27	3.86	4.61
	(1.41 to 1.60)	(1.95 to 2.25)	(2.28 to 2.71)	(1.40 to 1.64)	(2.25 to 2.64)	(2.61 to 3.25)	(2.07 to 2.48)	(3.50 to 4.26)	(4.32 to 5.36)
Housework									
Never	Ref	Ref	Ref	Ref	Ref	Ref	Ref	Ref	Ref
Sometimes	1.42	1.65	1.44	1.46	1.76	1.70	1.79	2.21	2.05
	(1.35 to 1.50)	(1.56 to 1.76)	(1.33 to 1.56)	(1.36 to 1.56)	(1.64 to 1.89)	(1.54 to 1.87)	(1.66 to 1.93)	(2.04 to 2.39)	(1.87 to 2.24)
Often	1.32	1.79	2.11	1.31	2.04	2.34	1.82	2.86	3.35
	(1.25 to 1.40)	(1.68 to 1.90)	(1.95 to 2.28)	(1.22 to 1.40)	(1.89 to 2.19)	(2.13 to 2.58)	(1.68 to 1.96)	(2.62 to 3.11)	(3.05 to 3.67)
Daily travel									
Never	Ref	Ref	Ref	Ref	Ref	Ref	Ref	Ref	Ref
Sometimes	1.36	1.60	1.36	1.40	1.66	1.51	1.64	2.00	1.78
	(1.28 to 1.44)	(1.49 to 1.70)	(1.25 to 1.49)	(1.30 to 1.50)	(1.54 to 1.79)	(1.35 to 1.67)	(1.52 to 1.77)	(1.84 to 2.18)	(1.61 to 1.97)
Often	1.33	1.82	2.13	1.36	2.13	2.30	1.85	2.82	3.51
	(1.26 to 1.41)	(1.72 to 1.94)	(1.97 to 2.30)	(1.28 to 1.46)	(1.98 to 2.28)	(2.10 to 2.53)	(1.71 to 1.99)	(2.60 to 3.06)	(3.21 to 3.85)
Work									
Never	Ref	Ref	Ref	Ref	Ref	Ref	Ref	Ref	Ref
Sometimes	1.32	1.63	1.40	1.40	1.65	1.64	1.78	2.22	2.08
	(1.24 to 1.40)	(1.52 to 1.75)	(1.28 to 1.54)	(1.30 to 1.51)	(1.52 to 1.80)	(1.46 to 1.84)	(1.63 to 1.93)	(2.03 to 2.44)	(1.87 to 2.32)
Often	1.37	1.87	2.17	1.36	2.13	2.45	1.85	2.96	3.64
	(1.30 to 1.45)	(1.75 to 1.99)	(2.01 to 2.36)	(1.27 to 1.45)	(1.98 to 2.29)	(2.22 to 2.71)	(1.71 to 1.99)	(2.73 to 3.24)	(3.31 to 4.00)
Exercise									
Never	Ref	Ref	Ref	Ref	Ref	Ref	Ref	Ref	Ref
Sometimes	1.26	1.40	1.10	1.41	1.58	1.33	1.57	1.90	1.55
	(1.19 to 1.33)	(1.32 to 1.48)	(1.02 to 1.18)	(1.32 to 1.51)	(1.48 to 1.70)	(1.21 to 1.46)	(1.45 to 1.71)	(1.75 to 2.05)	(1.42 to 1.69)
Often	1.17	1.42	1.38	1.24	1.59	1.57	1.58	2.16	2.14
	(1.11 to 1.24)	(1.33 to 1.51)	(1.28 to 1.49)	(1.16 to 1.33)	(1.48 to 1.71)	(1.43 to 1.73)	(1.46 to 1.71)	(1.98 to 2.35)	(1.94 to 2.35)

*Multivariate regression adjusting for potential confounders: age, sex, marital status, work status, household income, urban-rural residence, exercise, housework, hours of sleep, body mass index, smoking and drinking.
†Life satisfaction scores: highest=9–10, high=8, medium=6–7 and low=0–5.

Tawatsupa B, Yiengprugsawan V, Kjellstrom T, et al. BMJ Open 2012;2:e001396. doi:10.1136/bmjopen-2012

er motivation to work and experienced more nega-
moods in hot environments. Anderson found that
prolonged, continuous repetitive actions required to
intain performance at work and achieve target goals
ch as getting a job finished) can lead to hyperten-
n.[32] And when more effort was required to complete
ask in hot conditions loss of motivation was experi-
ed leading to lower productivity and increased injury
. The impact of heat stress on psychological perform-
e variables[11] is a likely factor in these work-related
acts of heat.
sychological effects of heat stress have been noted in
er settings as well. Nitschke et al[33] reported a positive
ociation between high-ambient temperature and hos-
l admissions for mental and behavioural disorders in
laide, Australia. Specific illnesses for which admis-
s increased included anxiety, symptomatic mood dis-
ers and psychological development disorders among
erly people when temperature exceeded 26.7°C.[34]
reover, excessive heat stress exposure may also
ease violence.[32-35] Increasing heat stress had been
ociated with higher rates of aggressive behaviour,[36]
higher violent suicide rates.[37] In a meta-analysis,
chama et al[38] concluded that pre-existing mental
lth problems tripled the risk of all-cause mortality
ing a heat wave. A related issue is the physical and
hological exhaustion caused by extreme heat stress.[7]
our study, we found that heat stress in Thailand is
only a problem at work but also heat stress interferes
other daily activities including sleeping, daily travel,
sework and exercise. The results of our study com-
nent other Thai research about adverse effects of
. One recent report shows that heat stress in
iland is a very serious problem in a wide variety of
settings.[18] McMichael et al[19] and Guo et al[39] found
mperature–mortality association and Pudpong and
t[20] found heat-related excess hospital admissions.
ker studies in Thailand related occupational heat
s, kidney disease and psychological distress.[10 21]
he limitation of this study is that it could not directly
lish that health and well-being outcomes arose as a
lt of heat stress. Interpreting causality between heat
s exposure and health and well-being outcomes is
plex in a cross-sectional study as we cannot be com-
ly sure that heat stress preceded their health condi-
and well-being. Also, the source of the heat stress
not reported and we could not make direct measure-
ts of heat stress exposure and health and well-being
omes. Another limitation of this study arose because
le answered the questionnaire at different times of
ear (but most in March–July—the hot period). The
tions on physical and emotional health assessed the
ous 4 weeks so most (almost all) were answering for
ot period.
e strength of this study is its large scale with partici-
n from a national group of adults embedded in the
economic mainstream of Thai society. Other

strengths include the comprehensive questionnaire
which captures a detailed assessment of health and an
array of geodemographic, environmental and social attributes. Also, the cohort has been set up for future longitudinal analysis which will provide better insight into
causal pathways between heat stress and subsequent
health outcomes in the long run.

We conclude that Thai populations are at high risk of
heat stress during daily activities. Also, in Thailand an
anticipated increase in temperature from climate
change plus the ageing and urbanisation of the population could significantly increase heat impacts on health
and well-being. There is a need for improvements in
public health surveillance and public awareness regarding the risks of heat stress which hitherto have been considered unremarkable in such a tropical environment.

Author affiliations
[1]National Centre for Epidemiology and Population Health, ANU College of
Medicine, Biology and Environment, the Australian National University,
Canberra, Australia
[2]Health Impact Assessment Division, Department of Health, Ministry of Public
Health, Nonthaburi, Thailand
[3]Centre for Global Health Research, Umeå University, Umeå, Sweden
[4]School of Human Ecology, Sukhothai Thammathirat Open University,
Nonthaburi, Thailand

Acknowledgements We thank the staff at Sukhothai Thammathirat Open
University (STOU) who assisted with student contact, and the STOU students
who are participating in the cohort study. We also thank Dr Bandit Thinkamrop
and his team from Khon Kaen University for guiding us successfully through the
complex data processing.

Collaborators Thailand: Jaruwan Chokhanapitak, Chaiyun Churewong,
Suttanit Hounthasarn, Suwanee Khamman, Daoruang Pandee, Suttinan
Pangsap, Tippawan Prapamontol, Janya Puengson, Yodyiam Sangrattanakul,
Sam-ang Seubsman, Boonchai Somboonsook, Nintita Sripaiboonkij,
Pathumvadee Somsamai, Duangkae Vilainerun and Wanee
Wimonwattanaphan. Australia: Chris Bain, Emily Banks, Cathy Banwell, Bruce
Caldwell, Gordon Carmichael, Tarie Dellora, Jane Dixon, Sharon Friel, David
Harley, Matthew Kelly, Tord Kjellstrom, Lynette Lim, Roderick McClure,
Anthony McMichael, Tanya Mark, Adrian Sleigh, Lyndall Strazdins and
Vasoontara Yiengprugsawan.

Contributors The corresponding author had full access to all data used in the
study and had final responsibility for the decision to submit for publication. BT
and VY conceptualised the analysis for this paper with contributions from all
authors. BT and VY did the literature search and VY did
statistical analyses. TK had the initial idea for the heat stress study. SS and AS
conceived and executed the Thai Cohort Study and assisted with the writing and
interpretation. All authors contributed to and approved the final version.

Funding The International Collaborative Research Grants Scheme with joint
grants from the Wellcome Trust UK (GR071587MA) and the Australian
National Health and Medical Research Council (NHMRC 268055), and as a
global health grant from the NHMRC (585426).

Competing interests None.

Ethics approval Sukhothai Thammathirat Open University Research and
Development Institute (protocol 0522/10) and the Australian National
University Human Research Ethics Committee (protocol 2009/570).

Provenance and peer review Not commissioned; externally peer reviewed.

Data sharing statement Statistical code in Stata, and dataset available from
the corresponding author at ben_5708@hotmail.com. All Participants gave
informed consent and the presented data in this manuscript are anonymous.

REFERENCES

1. Confalonieri U, Menne B, Akhtar R, et al. Human health. Climate change 2007: impacts, adaptation and vulnerability. contribution of working group II to the fourth assessment report of the intergovernmental panel on climate change. Cambridge, UK: Cambridge University Press, 2007 (cited 13 March 2012); http://www.ipcc-wg2.org (accessed 13 March 2012).
2. Basu R, Samet JM. Relation between elevated ambient temperature and mortality: a review of the epidemiologic evidence. Epidemiol Rev 2002;24:190–202.
3. Kovats RS, Hajat S. Heat stress and public health: a critical review. Annu Rev Public Health 2008;29:41–55.
4. Basu R. High ambient temperature and mortality: a review of epidemiologic studies from 2001 to 2008. Environ Health 2009;8:40.
5. Bi P, Williams S, Loughnan M, et al. The effects of extreme heat on human mortality and morbidity in Australia: implications for public health. Asia Pac J Public Health 2011;23(2 Suppl):27S—36S.
6. Campbell-Lendrum D, Corvalan C. Climate change and developing-country cities: implications for environmental health and equity. J Urban Health 2007;84(1 Suppl):i109–17.
7. Parsons K. Human thermal environments: the effects of hot, moderate, and cold environments on human health, comfort and performance. 2nd edn. London: Taylor & Francis, 2003.
8. Kjellstrom T. Climate change, direct heat exposure, health and well-being in low and middle-income countries. Glob Health Action 2009;2:1–3.
9. Berry HL, Bowen K, Kjellstrom T. Climate change and mental health: a causal pathways framework. Int J Public Health 2010;55:123–32.
10. Tawatsupa B, Lim LL-Y, Kjellstrom T, et al. The association between overall health, psychological distress, and occupational heat stress among a large national cohort of 40 913 Thai workers. Glob Health Action 2010;3:1–10.
11. Hancock PA, Ross JM, Szalma JL. A meta-analysis of performance response under thermal stressors. Hum Factors 2007;49:851–77.
12. Kjellstrom T. Climate change exposures, chronic disease and mental health in urban populations:a threat to health security, particularly for the poor and disadvantaged. Kobe, Japan: World Health Organization Centre for Health and Development, 2009.
13. Kjellstrom T, Holmer I, Lemke B. Workplace heat stress, health and productivity—an increasing challenge for low and middle-income countries during climate change. Glob Health Action 2009;2:1–6.
14. Kjellstrom T, Gabrysch S, Lemke B, et al. The 'Hothaps' program for assessing climate change impacts on occupational health and productivity: an invitation to carry out field studies. Glob Health Action 2009;2:1–7.
15. Tawatsupa B, Dear K, Kjellstrom T, et al. The association between temperature and mortality in tropical middle income Thailand from 1999 to 2008. Int J Biometeorol 2012:1–13.
16. Limsakul A, Goes JI. Empirical evidence for interannual and longer period variability in Thailand surface air temperatures. Atmos Res 2008;87:89–102.
17. Thai Meteorological Department. Climate change in Thailand for last 52 years. Bangkok: Meteorological Department, Thailand, 2007. http://www.tmd.go.th/info/info.php?FileID=86 (accessed 4 Feb 2012).
18. Langkulsen U, Vichit-Vadakan N, Taptagaporn S. Health impact of climate change on occupational health and productivity in Thailand. Glob Health Action 2010;3:1–9.
19. McMichael AJ, Wilkinson P, Kovats RS, et al. International st temperature, heat and urban mortality: the 'ISOTHURM' proj Epidemiol 2008;37:1121–31.
20. Pudpong N, Hajat S. High temperature effects on out-patien and hospital admissions in Chiang Mai, Thailand. Sci Total 2011;409:5260–7.
21. Tawatsupa B. Lim LL-Y, Kjellstrom T, et al. Association betw occupational heat stress and kidney disease among 37 816 workers in the Thai Cohort Study (TCS). J Epidemiol 2012;22:251–60.
22. Sleigh A, Seubsman S, Bain C. Cohort profile: the Thai Coh of 87 134 Open University students. Int J Epidemiol 2008;37:266–72.
23. Grad FP. The preamble of the constitution of the World Hea Organization. Bull World Health Organ 2002;80:981–4.
24. Cummins RA, Eckersley R, Pallant J, et al. Developing a na index of subjective wellbeing: the Australian Unity Wellbeing Soc Indic Res 2003;64:159–90.
25. Yiengprugsawan V, Seubsman S, Khamman S, et al. Perso wellbeing index in a national cohort of 87 134 Thai adults. S Res 2010;98:201–15.
26. StataCorp. Stata 12.0 for windows. College Station, TX: StataCorporation, 2011.
27. Kanazawa M, Yoshiike N, Osaka T, et al. Criteria and classi of obesity in Japan and Asia-Oceania. Asia Pac J Clin Nutr S732–7.
28. Hajat S, O'Connor M, Kosatsky T. Health effects of hot wea from awareness of risk factors to effective health protection. 2010;375:856–63.
29. McMichael AJ, Woodruff RE, Hales S. Climate change and health: present and future risks. Lancet 2006;367:859–69.
30. Kjellstrom T, Butler AJ, Lucas RM, et al. Public health impac of global heating due to climate change: potential effects on chronic non-communicable diseases. Int J Public Health 2010;55:97–103.
31. Lan L, Lian Z, Pan L. The effects of air temperature on offic workers' well-being, workload and productivity-evaluated wit subjective ratings. Appl Ergon 2010;42:29–36.
32. Anderson C. Heat and violence. Curr Dir Psychol Sci 2001;
33. Nitschke M, Tucker GR, Bi P. Morbidity and mortality during heatwaves in metropolitan Adelaide. Med J Aust 2007;187:6
34. Hansen AL, Bi P, Nitschke M, et al. The effect of heat wave mental health in a temperate Australian city. Environ Health Perspect 2008;116:1369–75.
35. Anderson C, Anderson K, Dorr N, et al. Temperature and aggression. Adv Exp Soc Psychol 2000;32:63–133.
36. Cheatwood D. The effects of weather on homicide. J Quant 1995;11:51–70.
37. Maes M, De Meyer F, Thompson P, et al. Synchronized anr rhythms in violent suicide rate, ambient temperature and the light-dark span. Acta Psychiatr Scand 1994;90:391–6.
38. Bouchama A, Dehbi M, Mohamed G, et al. Prognostic facto wave-related deaths: a meta-analysis. Arch Intern Med 2007;167:2170–6.
39. Guo Y, Punnasiri K, Tong S. Effects of temperature on mort Chiang Mai city, Thailand: a time series study. Environ Heal 2012;11:36.

Tawatsupa B, Yiengprugsawan V, Kjellstrom T, et al. BMJ Open 2012;2:e001396. doi:10.1136/bmjopen-2012

Heat stress, health and well-being: findings from a large national cohort of Thai adults

Benjawan Tawatsupa, Vasoontara Yiengprugsawan, Tord Kjellstrom, et al.

BMJ Open 2012 2:
doi: 10.1136/bmjopen-2012-001396

Updated information and services can be found at:
http://bmjopen.bmj.com/content/2/6/e001396.full.html

These include:

References	This article cites 33 articles, 5 of which can be accessed free at: http://bmjopen.bmj.com/content/2/6/e001396.full.html#ref-list-1
Open Access	This is an open-access article distributed under the terms of the Creative Commons Attribution Non-commercial License, which permits use, distribution, and reproduction in any medium, provided the original work is properly cited, the use is non commercial and is otherwise in compliance with the license. See: http://creativecommons.org/licenses/by-nc/2.0/ and http://creativecommons.org/licenses/by-nc/2.0/legalcode.
Email alerting service	Receive free email alerts when new articles cite this article. Sign up in the box at the top right corner of the online article.

Topic Collections	Articles on similar topics can be found in the following collections Epidemiology (286 articles) Occupational and environmental medicine (59 articles) Public health (258 articles)

Notes

CHAPTER 7: HEAT STRESS AND MORTALITY[5]

The chapter presents the association between weather variability and age-sex adjusted death rates (ADRs) in Thailand over a 10 year period from 1999 to 2008. Mortality, population, weather and air pollution datasets were obtained from four national databases. Multivariable Fractional Polynomial regression models (MFP) and multivariable linear regression models were developed in sequence to explore the associations between weather variation and deaths. ADR is the health outcome and was directly standardised using the age-sex distribution for the Thai population. The association between ADRs and six weather variables (maximum temperature, mean temperature, minimum temperature, precipitation, dew point temperature, and wind speed) are investigated. The effect of air pollution is later adjusted into the model. The associations are explored and compared among three seasons (cold, hot and wet months) and four weather zones of Thailand - the North (mountain area), the Northeast (subtropical and inland tropical area), the South (equatorial area), and the Central including Bangkok (tropical and urban area). The results of this chapter are useful for health impact assessment for the present situation and for estimating the future public health implications of global climate change.

---

[5] A version of Chapter 7 has been published. Tawatsupa B, Dear K, Kjellstrom T, Sleigh A (2012) The association between temperature and mortality in tropical middle income Thailand from 1999 to 2008. *International Journal of Biometeorology* (ICB 2011-Students/new professionals). DOI: 10.1007/s00484-012-0597-8

Int J Biometeorol
DOI 10.1007/s00484-012-0597-8

The association between temperature and mortality in tropical middle income Thailand from 1999 to 2008

Benjawan Tawatsupa · Keith Dear · Tord Kjellstrom · Adrian Sleigh

Received: 30 May 2012 / Revised: 3 October 2012 / Accepted: 3 October 2012
© ISB 2012

Abstract We have investigated the association between tropical weather condition and age-sex adjusted death rates (ADR) in Thailand over a 10-year period from 1999 to 2008. Population, mortality, weather and air pollution data were obtained from four national databases. Alternating multivariable fractional polynomial (MFP) regression and stepwise multivariable linear regression analysis were used to sequentially build models of the associations between temperature variable and deaths, adjusted for the effects and interactions of age, sex, weather (6 variables), and air pollution (10 variables). The associations are explored and compared among three seasons (cold, hot and wet months) and four weather zones of Thailand (the North, Northeast, Central, and South regions). We found statistically significant associations between temperature and mortality in Thailand.

The maximum temperature is the most important variable in predicting mortality. Overall, the association is nonlinear U-shape and 31 °C is the minimum-mortality temperature in Thailand. The death rates increase when maximum temperature increase with the highest rates in the North and Central during hot months. The final equation used in this study allowed estimation of the impact of a 4 °C increase in temperature as projected for Thailand by 2100; this analysis revealed that the heat-related deaths will increase more than the cold-related deaths avoided in the hot and wet months, and overall the net increase in expected mortality by region ranges from 5 to 13 % unless preventive measures were adopted. Overall, these results are useful for health impact assessment for the present situation and future public health implication of global climate change for tropical Thailand.

Keywords Climate change · Temperature · Mortality · Thailand · Tropical

Electronic supplementary material The online version of this article (doi:10.1007/s00484-012-0597-8) contains supplementary material, which is available to authorized users.

The article was made as preparation for publication in a Special Issue of International Journal of Biometeorology (IJB).

B. Tawatsupa
Health Impact Assessment Division, Department of Health,
Ministry of Public Health,
Nonthaburi, Thailand

B. Tawatsupa (✉) · K. Dear · T. Kjellstrom · A. Sleigh
National Centre for Epidemiology and Population Health,
ANU College of Medicine, Biology and Environment,
The Australian National University,
0200, Canberra, ACT, Australia
e-mail: ben_5708@hotmail.com

T. Kjellstrom
Centre for Global Health Research, Umeå University,
Umeå, Sweden

Introduction

For the last two decades interest in the impact of climate change on human health has grown. Several researchers have studied temperature-related mortality and found significant association between temperature and deaths (Kunst et al. 1993; Martens 1998; Braga et al. 2001; Armstrong 2006). These studies focused on the effects of temperature on mortality using various designs. Many studies adopted a time series approach (Stafoggia et al. 2009; Gasparrini and Armstrong 2010; Gasparrini et al. 2011; Guo et al. 2012). Several researchers used a case-crossover study design (Stafoggia et al. 2006; Tong et al. 2010) and some studies focused on extreme events such as heat waves in the United

States, Europe, Australia, and China (Baccini et al. 2008; Anderson and Bell 2009; D'Ippoliti et al. 2010; Khalaj et al. 2010; Liu and Zhang 2010).

Most studies on temperature-mortality associations have been conducted in temperate developed countries. They leave unanswered questions about the effects of warmer and humid weather in tropical countries where very high heat will become even more frequent under global climate change. Also, populations with limited adaptive capacity who live in developing countries where air pollution is already a problem may have worse health impacts from exposure to high temperatures (McMichael et al. 1998; Patz et al. 2005).

Thailand is a tropical and developing country with around one third of its population located in urban areas (National Statistical Office 2008). Climate change and its expected health effects in Thailand have received little attention. There have been very few studies on association between heat and health impacts in Thailand and they covered only two cities—Bangkok and Chiang Mai (McMichael et al. 2008; Pudpong and Hajat 2011; Guo et al. 2012)—or were restricted to a large national cohort of adult workers (Tawatsupa et al. 2010, 2012). McMichael et al. (2008) and Guo et al. (2012) found the non-linear relationship between daily mean temperature and non-external deaths. Pudpong and Hajat (2011) found heat-related excess hospital admissions. The worker studies related occupational heat stress, kidney disease and psychological distress (Tawatsupa et al. 2010, 2012).

Global warming is expected to increase future heat deaths. Average temperature in Thailand has increased 0.74 °C over the last century (Limsakul et al. 2009). From 1951 to 2003, the monthly mean maximum temperature in Thailand increased by 0.56 °C and the monthly mean minimum temperature increased even more by 1.44 °C (Limsakul and Goes 2008). Increasing heat stress is anticipated as Thailand urbanizes because of the urban heat island effect together with global warming (Taniguchi 2006). Also, existing air pollution will potentially interact with heat effects, with heat making the air pollution worse, and both contributing to excess mortality.

As already mentioned, little is known of the effect of temperature on mortality in a tropical environment. Furthermore, the interaction of tropical heat, urbanisation and air pollution as health risk factors is complex and little understood. To address this important gap in our knowledge, we investigated the relationship between weather condition, air pollution and total mortality in tropical Thailand during the period 1999 to 2008.

Materials and methods

To analyse the association between weather condition and mortality in Thailand we used four national databases. These covered 1999 to 2008 and included data on mid-year populations, mortality, weather, and air pollution, as described below.

Population data

The Ministry of Public Health, Thailand supplied mid-year populations by age-group and sex for each of Thailand's 76 provinces from 1999 to 2008 (Bureau of Policy and Strategy 2010b). These population data allowed the calculation of age-sex specific death rates for each province.

Mortality data

The Ministry of Public Health supplied daily all-cause mortality data for Thailand's 76 provinces (a total 3,805,638 deaths) from the 1st of January 1999 to the 31st of December 2008 (Bureau of Policy and Strategy 2010a). Outlier data (unusually high or low daily death counts in a province) were defined as being six standard deviations above or below the provincial mean daily death count for the entire 10-year period. Daily data that were so exceptional were deleted. This removed anomalous high death counts due to natural disasters (e.g. Indian Ocean Tsunami on December 26, 2004). It also removed anomalous low death counts due to end-of-year transfer of records to New Year registers.

For each province, daily death counts were averaged each month and then divided by the actual population for each of 18 age-sex groups to calculate monthly age-sex death rates across the 10 years. Each year, these actual provincial monthly age-sex death rates were then weighted and adjusted to the average age-sex structure for the whole of Thailand and updated annually (the formula is in Supplementary Material 1). This adjustment corrects the number of deaths observed in each of 76 provinces to estimate deaths that would have occurred (per 100,000) with a standard age-sex structure.

Weather data

The Meteorological Department, Ministry of Information and Communication Technology supplied daily weather data for a total of 120 stations in 65 provinces from 1999 to 2008 (Meteorological Development Bureau 2010). The daily weather data include six weather variables for calculating monthly weather profiles of Thailand: mean, minimum, maximum and average dew point temperatures (°C), maximum wind speed (m/s), and average precipitation in 24 h (mm). We also had measurements of the relative humidity but we did not use them in the first set of models because of collinearity with the related measure of dew point temperature (i.e. variance inflation factor [VIF]>9). We did use relative humidity in later models that did not include dew point temperature (see sensitivity analysis section below).

Air pollution data

The Pollution Control Department, Ministry of Natural Resources and Environment, supplied the air pollution data for 23 provinces with fixed air quality monitoring stations (Air Quality and Noise Management Bureau 2010). The monthly maximum and monthly average of daily mean concentrations for five air pollutants are used in this study: 1-h average of sulphur dioxide (SO_2), 1-h average of nitrogen dioxide (NO_2), 1-h average of carbon monoxide (CO), 1-h average of ozone (O_3), and 24-h average of particulate matter of less than 10 μm in diameter (PM_{10}).

Statistical analysis

We assume that weather and air pollution exposure are uniform within provinces. Some provinces have more than one weather station or more than one air quality monitoring station but the monthly fluctuations are very similar. Therefore, for each province, we calculated monthly averages of daily weather and air pollution data of each station, and then used the simple average of monthly weather and air pollution data from all stations in that province as the provincial monthly weather and air pollution condition. The weather-mortality analyses are divided into three phases as follows (Fig. 1): developing weather-mortality models, selecting the best weather model for adding air pollution effects, and assessing weather models adjusted for air pollution effects. For the first phase, models A to E were sequentially developed to test the links between weather and mortality based on the data for 53 provinces with complete weather and death datasets (N=5,599 province-months). Then for the second phase we selected the best weather model from phase one (model D). For the third phase we restricted analysis to 13 provinces with weather, air pollution and death datasets (N=1,025 province-months). Starting with model D we added air-pollution adjustments to create models F1 to F4. We produced an optimal weather-death model adjusted for air pollution effects (model F4). We used this model to estimate expected mortality with a 4 °C increase in temperature as projected for Thailand by 2100.

Developing models to test the links between weather and mortality

The main question of interest was how the monthly mortality (adjusted death rates [ADR] per 100,000 population) related to weather condition. The dependent variable was monthly provincial ADR from 1999 to 2008. Explanatory monthly provincial weather data were included if they were available for all six weather variables—mean, minimum,

maximum and dew point temperatures, wind speed, and precipitation.

Each of the six weather variables from the 5,599 province-months were aggregated and checked for distribution skewness and unduly influential values. Four of the six weather variables had approximately normal distributions but wind speed and precipitation were very positively skewed. To reduce the undue influence of skewed high values in regression models we converted the distributions of wind speed and precipitation using an optimal transformation (Stata 2011). We chose log-transformation ($\ln(x+1)$) of wind speed and precipitation, with plus one added to avoid the problem of zero transforms, as this produced the most symmetrical distribution with no extreme values. These initial transformations improved the explanatory power of wind speed and precipitation and reduced the possibility of artefactual interactions in subsequent multi-variable fractional polynomial (MFP) models (Royston and Sauerbrei 2008).

MFP and linear regressions then were used with the statistical package Stata/SE12 (Stata 2011) to mathematically define relationships between deaths and weather variables and their interactions at a significance level of $p \leq 0.001$. MFP models devised optimal transformations for the raw (untransformed) weather variables and stepwise linear regression analyses selected the most significant explanatory variables produced by the MFP models. The results of the linear regression models were tested by R^2, function plots (graphs), and goodness of fit criteria developed by Akaike (1974). The Akaike's information criterion (AIC) identified the best model to fit the overall relationship between the weather variables and ADR. The alternating progressive application of increasingly complex MFP and linear regression produced 49 models in five sequential groups (models A to E).

The multivariable fractional polynomial (MFP) regression is suited to continuous, multivariable, non-linear associations (Royston and Sauerbrei 2008). It was developed by Royston and Altman (Cleves et al. 2008). Fractional polynomial models are intermediate between polynomial and nonlinear models. According to Royston and Sauerbrei (2008), a fractional polynomial of degree m with power $\boldsymbol{p} = (p_1, \ldots, p_m)$ is defined as:

$$FP(m) = \beta_1 X^{p_1} + \beta_2 X^{p_2} + \ldots + \beta_m X^{p_m} \qquad (1)$$

The objective of fractional polynomials is to obtain the best values of the degree m and of power $p_1, \ldots, p_m$ by comparing the deviances of different models. For a given m, the best-fitting powers $p_1, \ldots, p_m$ corresponding to the model with the smallest deviance are selected (Cleves et al. 2008).

Five equation formats (A to E) were used for the progressively more complex models linking weather and death rates

Fig. 1 Analysis sequence for
investigating relationship
between weather condition, air
pollution and deaths in
Thailand, 1999–2008

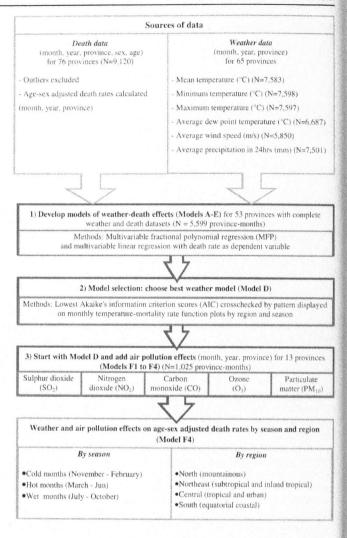

Sources of data	
Death data (month, year, province, sex, age) for 76 provinces (N=9,120)	*Weather data* (month, year, province) for 65 provinces
- Outliers excluded	- Mean temperature (°C) (N=7,583)
- Age-sex adjusted death rates calculated	- Minimum temperature (°C) (N=7,598)
(month, year, province)	- Maximum temperature (°C) (N=7,597)
	- Average dew point temperature (°C) (N=6,687)
	- Average wind speed (m/s) (N=5,850)
	- Average precipitation in 24hrs (mm) (N=7,501)

1) Develop models of weather-death effects (Models A-E) for 53 provinces with complete weather and death datasets (N = 5,599 province-months)
Methods: Multivariable fractional polynomial regression (MFP) and multivariable linear regression with death rate as dependent variable

2) Model selection: choose best weather model (Model D)
Methods: Lowest Akaike's information criterion scores (AIC) crosschecked by pattern displayed on monthly temperature-mortality rate function plots by region and season

3) Start with Model D and add air pollution effects (month, year, province) for 13 provinces **(Models F1 to F4)** (N=1,025 province-months)

Sulphur dioxide (SO₂)	Nitrogen dioxide (NO₂)	Carbon monoxide (CO)	Ozone (O₃)	Particulate matter (PM₁₀)

Weather and air pollution effects on age-sex adjusted death rates by season and region (Model F4)

By season	*By region*
●Cold months (November - February)	●North (mountainous)
●Hot months (March - Jun)	●Northeast (subtropical and inland tropical)
●Wet months (July - October)	●Central (tropical and urban)
	●South (equatorial coastal)

(Supplementary Material 2 describes the main characteristics of the models). The sequence of formats used was as follows.

Model A is a single MFP function with monthly deaths for Thailand as the dependent variable and significant transformed ("functional form") weather variables as the independent variables. Model A was adjusted for year (10 levels), month (12 levels), and province (65 provinces) as factor variables (1 model).

Model B is a set of 20 models that begins with an MFP of model A plus 15 transformed (functional form) pairwise interaction terms for the six weather variables (1 model); model B is then further developed using the same weather functional forms to perform a linear regression restricted by

region (4 models), by season (3 models), or by region-season interactions (12 models).

Model C is a set of 19 models, as an MFP of model B restricted by region (4 models), by season (3 models) or by region-season (12 models).

Model D is a set of four models (D1 to D4) that begins with linear regression of the optimal (transformed) functional form of maximum temperature (identified as a key variable in earlier models) along with month, year, and province (1 model). Then other (untransformed) weather variables are added to the equation (1 model), then untransformed weather variable interactions are also added (1 model). Finally, an MFP model of the independent variables from the previous model, with all weather and interaction variables converted to optimal functional forms, becomes the final model of the set.

Model E is a set of five models. The set begins with a linear regression of monthly deaths using as independent variables two functional forms of maximum temperature by region-season (1 model), then it adds the untransformed weather variables (1 model), and then adds the untransformed weather variable interactions (1 model). The previous (third) model in the set is then further transformed using MFP to convert all weather variables and their interactions into optimal function forms (1 model). The fourth model is then repeated by stepwise linear regression so that only statistically significant weather-related variables were included, along with month, year, and province (1 model).

Model selection criteria

We chose the models with the lowest (best) AIC scores and best fit for weather and mortality. As models A to E used different approaches, the decisions for selecting the best of these 49 models depended on the R^2 and the best goodness-of-fit using AIC. Optimal models also needed to be easily interpretable as graphical function plots. We chose model A (simple equation) and models D1 and D4 (complex equations). Model A shows why maximum temperature is the most important variable and model D4 incorporates transformed maximum temperature and many other explanatory weather variables to produce the most accurate equation linking mortality and weather.

Model A is a single MFP regression exploring the overall relationship between weather condition and mortality for the whole country but cannot separate by season or region. Model D is statistically the best model with the lowest AIC and clearly interpretable exposure-response curves for the temperature and mortality relationship for each region-season graph. Model D is therefore used in this report to show how maximum temperature relates to death rates across seasons and regions after adjusting with the six weather variables and their 15 interactions. Completion of models A to E, with analyses restricted to weather and mortality, prepared for the next stage involving addition of air pollution data. The air pollution models are now described.

Air pollution adjusted-models

To investigate potential modifier and confounding effects of air pollution, we gathered available air pollution data and explored the influence of air pollution on the weather-mortality effects revealed by models A to E. The ten air pollution variables are monthly average of daily mean and daily maximum concentrations of SO_2, NO_2, CO, O_3, PM_{10}. Some of the air pollution variables had values that included zero and overall their distributions were positively skewed.

To reduce the influence of extreme values, all the air pollution variables were log transformed with plus one to remove zeros ($\ln(x + 1)$). Missing values of air pollution variables in any month resulted in exclusion of that month from analysis.

Air pollution data were available in 13 provinces over 1,025 province-months (Fig. 2). These data were added to the D models to ascertain the influence of air pollution, a potential confounder of weather effects on mortality. So, an F set of four more models was created to enable analysis of air pollution effects; model F1 is a linear regression structurally identical to model D1 (adjusted for all weather variables without addition of air pollution variables); it is used as an F model benchmark to compare to the other F models that all include air pollution variables. These are linear regression models F2 to F4, and they are structurally identical to models D2 to D4 with the addition of the ten air pollution variables (maximum and mean SO_2, NO_2, CO, O_3, PM_{10}). Models F2 and F3 use untransformed weather and air pollution variables. Model F4 is an MFP model that transforms the weather, air pollution, and interaction variables into optimal functional forms. It enabled a series of season-region specific mortality function plots that displayed a "best-fit" for the mortality data. The function plots show the link between maximum temperature and change in ADR for each of the 12 season-region combinations. Each graph shows the magnitude of temperature effects on mortality and the optimum temperature for minimum mortality.

Climate change projections

For each region and each season in Thailand, we estimated the impacts of temperature increases. First we calculated the differences in ADR at the optimum temperature compared to the 90th percentile of maximum temperature. We also estimated the ADR expected with an additional 4 °C increase of maximum temperature, the increase projected for Thailand by 2100 (Thai Meteorological Department 2009).

Sensitivity analysis of results using other heat stress measures

To test the performance of two other heat stress measures that appear in the research literature we repeated the above sequence of 53 mortality models (model A to F) twice—once using wet bulb globe temperature (WBGT) (Gagge and Nishi 1976) and once for heat index (HI) (Steadman 1979). Both measures are complicated composites of maximum temperature and relative humidity—the formulas to create them are reproduced in Supplementary Material 1. These new sets of temperature-mortality models were adjusted for wind speed, rain and WBGT (one set) or wind speed, rain and heat index (one set). Results were similar to those generated by the first set of 53 models so the WBGT and HI results are not shown.

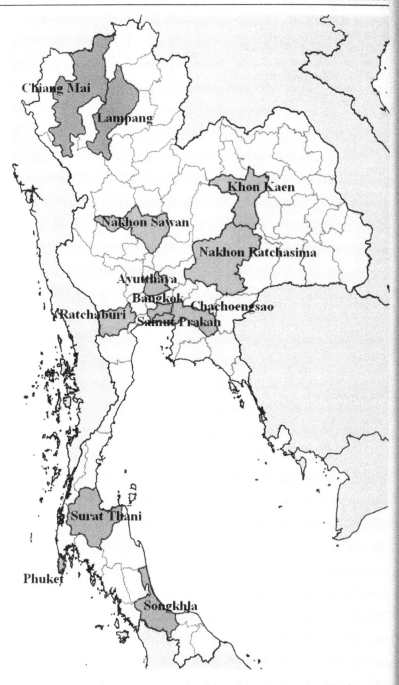

Fig. 2 Geographical variation of 13 provinces in final MFP model with air pollution effects (modified from http://commons.wikimedia.org/wiki/File:BlankMap_Thailand.png, by Ahoerstemeier, via Wikimedia Commons)

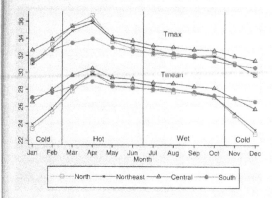

Fig. 3 Monthly average of mean and maximum temperatures by month and region ($N=5,599$ province-months)

Results

Weather conditions in Thailand

Overall, using available data for 53 provinces, the average maximum temperature, mean temperature and minimum temperature in degrees Celsius over the 10 years were 32.7, 27.4 and 22.5, respectively (Supplementary Material 3). Average monthly maximum and mean temperatures over 10 years are presented for each region in Fig. 3. The seasons are shown as hot months (March to June), wet months (July to October), and cold months (November to February). The maximum temperature averaged over the 10-year periods varied little by region (32.2–33.4 °C) (Supplementary Material 4). The North and Northeast region have temperature ranges wider than the South (Fig. 4). During 10 years, monthly maximum temperatures were highest in the North region during April (40.0 °C) and lowest in the same region during December (24.3 °C). The Central region commonly had high maximum temperature across the whole year, particularly in hot and wet months. Evidently, for maximum temperature effects on mortality, we need to compare results by season and region.

ADR trends in Thailand, 1999 to 2008

In the 53 Thai provinces with weather data available from 1999 to 2008 there were 2,754,848 deaths, an average of 22,957 per month over the 120 months observation. The average monthly provincial ADR during the 10 years was 50 deaths per 100,000 population with a range of 23.8 to 91.5 deaths per 100,000 population. The North had the highest average ADR at 53.9 per 100,000 population, followed by the Central region (51.2), the Northeast (49.4), and the South (46.1).

Association between mortality and weather in Thailand overall from 1999 to 2008

Model A The (full MFP) model of provincial ADR produced the optimal fitted function for each of the weather variables selected as significant at the 0.001 level. Maximum temperature, mean temperature, and precipitation were the most explanatory of ADR and were included in model A; the other three weather variables (minimum temperature, dew point temperature, and wind speed) were discarded ($p>0.001$). Model A accounts for 75 % of the variation in ADR ($R^2=0.75$). The deaths show marked nonlinearity for maximum temperature. Results from model A also showed that maximum temperature had the strongest weather variable influence on ADR. This influence was expressed ($p<0.001$) via the sum of two transformed terms of maximum temperature ($\beta_1 \text{Tmax}_1 + \beta_2 \text{Tmax}_2$), where

$$\text{Tmax}_1 = (\text{Tmax}/10)^3$$

$$\text{Tmax}_2 = (\text{Tmax}/10)^{3\,*}\ln(\text{Tmax}/10)$$

The polynomial plot of ADR by the functional maximum temperature terms is displayed in Fig. 5. Fluctuation of the maximum temperature in Thailand during the last 10 years (1999 to 2008) across the temperature range of 24 to 40 °C produced substantial variation in mortality. There is a strongly significant nonlinear association between monthly maximum temperature and mortality ($p<0.001$). As the maximum temperature rises from 24 °C to 31 °C, ADR exponentially falls; but when maximum temperature rises further, ADR exponentially increases. This crude analysis, averaged across 53 of Thailand's 76 provinces, indicates that 31 °C is the average optimum maximum temperature in Thailand.

Association between mortality, weather and air pollution by region-season

The association between mortality and weather condition shown above (Fig. 5) derived from data spanning 5,599 province-months from 53 provinces from 1999 to 2008. The mortality-weather association also needs to reflect the influences of geographical regions (tropical vs equatorial, inland vs coastal, plus urban heat island) and seasons (hot, wet, cold). Air pollution effects need to be analysed as well because they are likely to interact or confound the weather effects on mortality. Accordingly, our analyses consider various influential combinations of the weather variables along with geographical, seasonal, and air pollution effects in a final set of F models (see below). Monthly average values of weather and

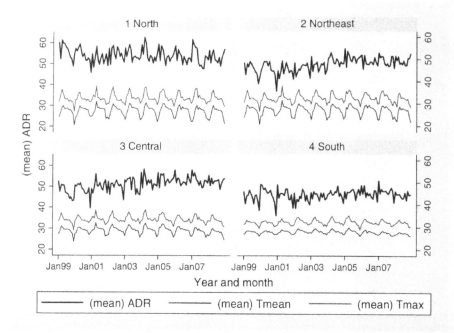

Fig. 4 Monthly variations of mortality rates against mean and maximum temperature across 10 years ($N=5{,}599$ province-months)

air pollution variables by regions are shown in Supplementary Material 5. However, these data for both weather and air pollution are somewhat restricted, available for only 13 provinces over 1,025 province-months. Overall, for the 13 provinces with air pollution and weather data, the hottest and most polluted area was the Central region.

We selected the model F set for final analyses as its models had the lowest AICs. Since maximum temperature in the two

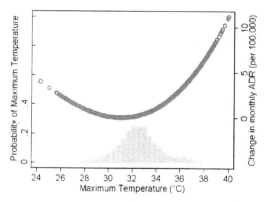

Fig. 5 Polynomial plot linking maximum temperature function (model A) to change in ADR and temperature density distribution in Thailand 1999–2008 ($N=5{,}599$ province-months)

functional forms used in models A, B, and C had the strongest influence, those two functional forms of maximum temperature were investigated as a main risk factor in all the models F set. One functional form is the cube of Tmax/10. The other functional form is the cube of Tmax/10 multiplied by the natural logarithm of Tmax/10. Models F1 to F4 explore the association between maximum temperature and mortality for each region and season, adjusting for air pollution. Thus, models F1 to F4 each produced 12 region-by-season regression coefficients of maximum temperature. The adjusted model (model F4; Fig. 6) shows J- or U-shaped associations between maximum temperature and mortality in all regions. The steep slopes are found in the North, Northeast, and Central regions—at high maximum temperature during hot months and at low maximum temperature in the cold months. The patterns in the South show much less variation of both mortality and temperature.

F4 was selected as the final model because it had the lowest AIC scores and a strongly significant association between maximum temperature and ADR ($p<0.001$). Furthermore, model F4 improved prediction of ADR (R^2 of model F1 was 0.73 and of model F4 was 0.80).

The non-linear function of maximum temperature in model F4 reveals the fully adjusted optimum temperature for low mortality among regions and seasons. There is little variation noted, especially in the equatorial South. Thus,

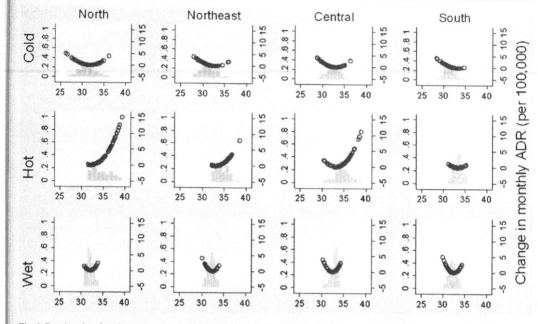

Fig. 6 Function plot of maximum temperature on ADR adjusted with air pollution, other weather variables and interactions by season and region plus temperature density distribution (final model F4) (*N*=1,025 province-months)

optimum temperatures in degrees Celsius in Thailand for low mortality range from 31.9 (North in the cold months) to 33.4 (South in the cold or hot months). In the wet season, optimum temperatures are similar for all regions, ranging from 32.2 to 32.5 °C.

This final F4 equation for linear regression and suitable functional transformations allowed modelling of the ADR for different maximum temperatures by region and season. Indeed, defining the optimum temperature for each region and each season allowed us to compare these ADRs to the region-season death rates expected at extreme hot temperatures (90th percentile of maximum temperature) (Table 1) and at additional 4 °C of maximum temperature as future climate projection in Thailand in 2100 (Thai Meteorological Department 2009) (Table 2). The largest difference in mortality in the future in relation to the 4 °C increase in maximum temperature is in the wet months leading to a net increase in ADR of 14 to 29 %, especially severe in the Central regions. The rising temperatures for the 4 °C scenario could reduce mortality rates during the cold months ranging from −1 to −8 %. Overall the net increase of mortality rates in the future for the full year of the 4 °C scenario ranged by region from 5 to 13 %. For the whole of Thailand the increase in mortality expected with a 4 °C increase in maximum temperature would be 8 %.

Discussion

We explored the association between weather and mortality in a tropical developing nation. This was done for 53 provinces in Thailand using 10 years of mortality data and parallel weather data. For 13 provinces, we were able to add air pollution data. Using a sequence of fractional polynomial regression and stepwise linear regression models we estimated the effect of temperature on mortality after adjusting for five other weather variables and ten pollution variables and the interactions. Overall 53 models were constructed and one final model was selected on statistical criteria. These 53 models were repeated for two other measures of heat stress (WBGT and HI) and the results for the temperature and mortality association were similar.

During the 10-year period analysed (1999–2008) there were highly significant associations between weather variation and mortality in Thailand. Out of six weather variables, maximum temperature was the most important in predicting mortality. When temperatures are lower or higher than optimum—which averaged 31 °C overall (53 provinces, model A)—the Thai mortality rate increases. After adding adjustments for air-pollution to model A and restricting to 13 provinces (ignoring region and season); we found that 33 °C was the optimum temperature.

For each region and season, the exposure-response curves present the association between maximum temperature and

Table 1 Percentage changes in optimal death rates (ADR) by changing maximum temperature to the 90th percentile, by region and season (final model F4)

Season	Region	Tmax (°C)		ADR[a] (deaths per 100,000)		
		Optimum Tmax	90th% Tmax	At optimum Tmax	At 90th % Tmax	% ADR differences
Cold	North	31.9	33.9	66.39	67.26	1.31
	Northeast	32.9	33.4	66.52	66.56	0.06
	Central	33.1	34.2	66.49	66.78	0.44
	South	33.4	32.6	66.42	66.55	0.19
Hot	North	32.1	37.6	66.45	74.96	12.81
	Northeast	33.0	36.3	66.51	69.25	4.12
	Central	33.1	36.6	66.48	70.28	5.71
	South	33.4	34.3	66.41	66.61	0.30
Wet	North	32.2	32.9	66.33	66.82	0.74
	Northeast	32.4	33.0	66.50	66.74	0.36
	Central	32.5	33.8	66.54	67.92	2.08
	South	32.5	33.5	66.55	67.25	1.05

[a] *ADR* monthly age-sex adjusted death rates

mortality rates as a J- or U-shape. Differences in slope of the temperature-mortality curve from region to region depend on weather conditions and the range of temperature to which the population has adapted (Iñiguez et al. 2010). The mortality-temperature graph has steep slopes at high maximum temperature in the hot months and at low maximum temperature in the cold months in the North, Northeast, and Central regions. In the presence of air pollution people are more sensitive to high maximum temperatures. Thus both weather and air pollution play a role in the

heat-mortality relationship (O'Neill et al. 2005; Iñiguez et al. 2010). We also compared the optimum temperature between adjusted and unadjusted air-pollution models (data not shown). The optimum temperatures in model F4 (adjusted for air pollution and their interactions) were a little bit lower (1 °C or less) than model F1 (unadjusted for air pollution) in all regions and seasons. The percent changes in the death rates by changing maximum temperature to the 90th percentile in model F4 are higher than model F1, especially during hot months in the North.

Table 2 Percentage changes in mortality rates (ADR) if maximum temperature were to increase 4°C[a], by region and season, and for overall Thailand (final model F4)

Season	Region	ADR[b] (deaths per 100,000)	ADR at Tmax +4°C[a]	Net changes in ADR	% change in ADR
Cold	North	62.57	61.12	−1.45	−2.32
	Northeast	51.52	48.70	−2.83	−5.49
	Central	55.36	54.79	−0.57	−1.03
	South	48.78	44.65	−4.13	−8.47
Hot	North	62.82	70.13	7.31	11.64
	Northeast	52.77	56.55	3.78	7.17
	Central	57.11	62.79	5.68	9.94
	South	49.36	50.09	0.73	1.48
Wet	North	60.60	69.24	8.64	14.26
	Northeast	50.88	58.67	7.79	15.31
	Central	56.31	72.44	16.13	28.64
	South	49.82	60.13	10.31	20.69
Overall	North	62.00	66.83	4.83	7.80
	Northeast	51.72	54.64	2.92	5.64
	Central	56.26	63.34	7.08	12.58
	South	49.34	51.89	2.56	5.18
	Thailand	54.98	59.39	4.41	8.01

[a] Expected temperature increase by 2100 for Thailand (see text)

[b] *ADR* monthly age-sex adjusted death rates

Strength and weakness of this study

The strengths of this study are the large national dataset for mortality, weather, and air pollution spanning 10 years obtained from various official sources. Weather condition and mortality rates were analysed across Thailand by seasons and regions adjusting for possible confounding by air pollution and its interactions. We found the weather and air pollution data used in this study were high-quality records which required minimal editing and were quite adequate for monthly averaging, a suitable technique in a stable climate like Thailand. One of us (BT) visited weather monitoring and air quality stations to assess the recording and reporting and was reassured by the dedication and training of the government officials involved.

The analysis used advanced statistical methods including non-linear multivariable fractional polynomial regression (MFP). The results are based on a series of 53 sequential MFP and linear regression models that enable detailed analysis of the temperature-mortality relationship. Furthermore, the final model permits estimate of the mortality outcomes if temperatures rise in Thailand. The model shows that the rising temperatures for the 4 °C scenario could reduce mortality rates during the cold months ranging from −1 to −8 %. However, the heat-related deaths will increase more than the cold-related deaths avoided in the hot and wet months and overall the net increase in expected mortality by region ranges from 5 to 13 %. For the whole of Thailand the increase in mortality expected with a 4 °C increase in maximum temperature would be 8 % unless humans adapt physiologically or adopt preventive behavior. Physiological adaptation is most unlikely and preventive behaviour is likely to be difficult to induce.

Comparison with other studies

Our findings associating high temperature and high population mortality are similar to other studies that investigate the relationship (Pan et al. 1995; Saez et al. 1995; Ballester et al. 1997; Keatinge et al. 2000; McMichael et al. 2008; Basu 2009; Iñiguez et al. 2010). The nonlinear temperature-mortality patterns we describe for tropical Thailand are similar to patterns reported for earlier temperate climate studies (Martens 1998; Armstrong 2006). However, the Thai population is adapted to higher temperatures than temperate climate residents as shown by the high optimum temperature exceeding 30 °C for lowest mortality in Thailand. The U- or J-shaped relationships between temperature and deaths occur in all regions of the world but the optimum temperature varies widely even within a relatively stable climate like tropical Thailand.

The weather variation between months in Thailand is relatively small compared to several other studies conducted in temperate countries (Bi et al. 2008). So the relationship found in this study needs to be compared with the results of other published literature in tropical and developing countries where hot weather has been associated with increased death rates such as heat waves in India and Bangladesh (Jendritzky 1999). Our national findings of a maximum temperature-mortality relationship demonstrate and quantify heat stress effects in tropical areas, and expand on two previous studies of Bangkok and Chiang Mai by McMichael et al. (2008) and Guo et al. (2012).

Guo et al. (2012) found a temperature-mortality association in Chiang Mai. McMichael et al. (2008) found large temperature effects on deaths in Bangkok, Chiang Mai and Mexico city, but mortality varied little across the narrow range of temperatures prevailing in San Salvador, due to its coastal location. In our study we found similar small changes in heat-related deaths and narrow ranges of temperature variation in the South of Thailand which is also located on an isthmus close to coastal areas and sea breezes.

Implications for public health

Maximum temperature is a useful indicator of heat exposure in health risk assessment and is easy to understand for cause-effect relationships. Many studies have found the relationship between mortality and maximum temperature has a U, V, or J shape (McMichael et al. 2008; Gosling et al. 2009). From our study maximum temperature can be used as an indicator for thermal stress of the population in Thailand. Maximum temperature monitoring would help public health surveillance of this risk and also be useful for health impact assessment of future climate change.

The results showed the largest effects of maximum temperature on mortality were in the inland tropical zones of Thailand. Unless the population is protected, global warming will increase the number of hot deaths and decrease the cold deaths in the Thai population. This will be especially prominent in urban areas due to heat island effects. If global warming extends to an increase of 4 °C (Thai Meteorological Department 2009), our findings suggest death rates will increase substantially especially in the hot and wet months of tropical inland zones, and this will affect much of Thailand.

Future research

Our study documents the adverse effect of high maximum temperature on the population in Thailand. For each region and season there are different optimum temperature and temperature-mortality slopes. However, the exact physical mechanisms and at risk subpopulations are unclear and further investigation is needed to determine who is actually dying and how high maximum temperatures are causing the deaths. Heat stress effects in different age groups are of particular interest especially mortality among working age groups (15–64 years) (Kjellstrom et al. 2009). The original report from the heat wave in France in August 2003 (Hémon and Jougla 2003)

documented almost 1000 additional deaths in the age range 20–60 years. This age group in still-not-rich Thailand is often exposed to heavy labour outdoors during hot weather most of the year (Tawatsupa et al. 2010, 2012). The elderly are also at high risk (Diaz et al. 2002; Basu et al. 2005; Hajat et al. 2007) and many of them are too poor to afford protective measures to avoid heat stress. Furthermore, the Thai population is aging and heat risks will steadily increase over time.

Acknowledgments We thank the staff at the Thai Meteorological Department, Ministry of Science and Technology (MOST), the Pollution Control Department, Ministry of Natural Resources and Environment (MONRE), and the Bureau of Policy and Strategy, Ministry of Public Health (MOPH), Thailand for providing the weather, air pollution, and mortality data used in this study. We also thank staff at the Department of Health, Thailand for their support throughout the study. Collaboration between ANU and Thailand underlying this study arose from the Thai Health-Risk Transition research project underway since 2004.

Ethical standards Ethics approval was obtained from the Australian National University Human Research Ethics Committee (protocol 2009/300).

Conflict of interest We declare that we have no conflict of interest. All authors contributed to and approved the final version of this manuscript.

References

Air Quality and Noise Management Bureau (2010) Daily air quality data. Pollution Control Department, Ministry of National Resources and Environment, Bangkok

Akaike H (1974) A new look at the statistical model identification. IEEE Trans Autom Control 19(6):716–723. doi:10.1109/TAC.1974.1100705.MR0423716

Anderson BG, Bell ML (2009) Weather-related mortality: how heat, cold, and heat waves affect mortality in the United States. Epidemiology 20(2):205–213. doi:10.1097/EDE.0b013e318190ee08

Armstrong B (2006) Models for the relationship between ambient temperature and daily mortality. Epidemiology 17(6):624–631. doi:10.1097/01.ede.0000239732.50999.8f

Baccini M, Biggeri A, Accetta G, Kosatsky T, Katsouyanni K, Analitis A, Anderson HR, Bisanti L, D'Ippoliti D, Danova J, Forsberg B, Medina S, Paldy A, Rabczenko D, Schindler C, Michelozzi P (2008) Heat effects on mortality in 15 European cities. Epidemiology 19(5):711–719. doi:10.1097/EDE.0b013e318176bfcd

Ballester F, Corella D, Perez-Hoyos S, Saez M, Hervas A (1997) Mortality as a function of temperature. A study in Valencia, Spain, 1991–1993. Int J Epidemiol 26(3):551–561. doi:10.1093/ije/26.3.551

Basu R (2009) High ambient temperature and mortality: a review of epidemiologic studies from 2001 to 2008. Environ Heal 8:40. doi:10.1186/1476-069X-8-40

Basu R, Dominici F, Samet JM (2005) Temperature and mortality among the elderly in the United States: a comparison of epidemiologic methods. Epidemiology 16(1):58–66. doi:10.1097/01.ede.0000147117.88386.fe

Bi P, Parton KA, Wang J, Donald K (2008) Temperature and direct effects on population health in Brisbane, 1986–1995. J Environ Health 70(8):48–53

Braga AL, Zanobetti A, Schwartz J (2001) The time course of weather-related deaths. Epidemiology 12(6):662–667

Bureau of Policy and Strategy (2010a) Daily mortality data. Office of Permanent Secretary, Ministry of Public Health, Nonthaburi

Bureau of Policy and Strategy (2010b) Number of mid-year population. Office of permanent Secretary, Ministry of Public Health, Nonthaburi

Cleves M, Gould W, Gutierrez R, Marchenko Y (2008) An introduction to survival analysis using Stata, 2nd edn. A Stata Press Publication, StataCorp LP, Texas

D'Ippoliti D, Michelozzi P, Marino C, De'Donato F, Menne B, Katsouyanni K, Kirchmayer U, Analitis A, Medina-Ramon M, Paldy A, Atkinson R, Kovats S, Bisanti L, Schneider A, Lefranc A, Iniguez C, Perucci CA (2010) The impact of heat waves on mortality in 9 European cities: results from the EuroHEAT project. Environmental Health 9:37. doi:10.1186/1476-069x-9-37

Diaz J, Garcia R, Velazquez de Castro F, Hernandez E, Lopez C, Otero A (2002) Effects of extremely hot days on people older than 65 years in Seville (Spain) from 1986 to 1997. Int J Biometeorol 46(3):145–149. doi:10.1007/s00484-002-0129-z

Gagge AP, Nishi Y (1976) Physical indices of the thermal environment. ASHRAE J 18(47–51)

Gasparrini A, Armstrong B (2010) Time series analysis on the health effects of temperature: advancements and limitations. Environ Res 110(6):633–638. doi:10.1016/j.envres.2010.06.005

Gasparrini A, Armstrong B, Kovats S, Wilkinson P (2011) The effect of high temperatures on cause-specific mortality in England and Wales. Occup Environ Med 69(1):56–61. doi:10.1136/oem.2010.059782

Gosling SN, Lowe JA, McGregor GR, Pelling M, Malamud BD (2009) Associations between elevated atmospheric temperature and human mortality: a critical review of the literature. Climate Change 92(3–4):299–341. doi:10.1007/s10584-008-9441-x

Guo Y, Punnasiri K, Tong S (2012) Effects of temperature on mortality in Chiang Mai city, Thailand: a time series study. Environ Heal 11(1):36. doi:10.1186/1476-069X-11-36

Hajat S, Kovats RS, Lachowycz K (2007) Heat-related and cold-related deaths in England and Wales: who is at risk? Occup Environ Med 64(2):93–100. doi:10.1136/oem.2006.029017

Hémon D, Jougla E (2003) Surmortalité liée à la canicule d'août 2003-Rapport d'étape. Estimation de la surmortalité et principales caractéristiques épidémiologiques [Excess mortality related to the heatwave of August 2003, Progress Report, Estimation of mortality and major epidemiological characteristics]. Institut National de la Santé et de la Recherche Médicale (INSERM) Paris, France

Iñiguez C, Ballester F, Ferrandiz J, Pérez-Hoyos S, Sáez M, López A, TEMPRO-EMECAS (2010) Relation between temperature and mortality in thirteen Spanish cities. Int J Environ Res Public Health 7:3196–3210. doi:10.3390/ijerph7083196

Jendritzky G (1999) Impacts of extreme and persistent temperatures— cold waves and heat waves. In: WMO/UNESCO sub-forum on sciance and technology in support of natural disaster reduction, Geneva. World Meteorological Organization, pp 43–52

Keatinge WR, Donaldson GC, Cordioli E, Martinelli M, Kunst AE, Mackenbach JP, Nayha S, Vuori I (2000) Heat related mortality in warm and cold regions of Europe: observational study. BMJ 321(7262):670–673. doi:10.1136/bmj.321.7262.670

Khalaj B, Lloyd G, Sheppeard V, Dear K (2010) The health impacts of heat waves in five regions of New South Wales, Australia: a case-only analysis. Int Arch Occup Environ Health 83(7):833–842. doi:10.1007/s00420-010-0534-2

Kjellstrom T, Holmer I, Lemke B (2009) Workplace heat stress, health and productivity—an increasing challenge for low and middle-income countries during climate change. Global Health Action 2. doi:DOI:10.3402/gha.v2i0.2047

Kunst AE, Looman CWN, Mackenbach JP (1993) Outdoor air temperature and mortality in The Netherlands: a time-series analysis. Am J Epidemiol 137(3):331–341

Limsakul A, Goes JI (2008) Empirical evidence for interannual and longer period variability in Thailand surface air temperatures. Atmos Res 87(2):89–102. doi:10.1016/j.atmosres.2007.07.007

Limsakul A, Limjirakan S, Sriburi T (2009) Trends in daily temperature extremes in Thailand. In: Ministry of Natural Resources and Environment (ed) Second National Conference on Natural Resources and Environment Bangkok, Thailand, p 59

Liu L, Zhang JL (2010) A case-crossover study between heat waves and daily death from cardiovascular and cerebrovascular disease. Zhonghua Liu Xing Bing Xue Za Zhi 31(2):179–184

Martens W (1998) Climate change, thermal stress and mortality changes. Soc Sci Med 46(3):331–344. doi:10.1016/S0277-9536(97)00162-7

McMichael AJ, Patz J, Kovats RS (1998) Impacts of global environmental change on future health and health care in tropical countries. Br Med Bull 54(2):475–488

McMichael AJ, Wilkinson P, Kovats RS, Pattenden S, Hajat S, Armstrong B, Vajanapoom N, Niciu EM, Mahomed H, Kingkeow C, Kosnik M, O'Neill MS, Romieu I, Ramirez-Aguilar M, Barreto ML, Gouveia N, Nikiforov B (2008) International study of temperature, heat and urban mortality: the 'ISOTHURM' project. Int J Epidemiol 37(5):1121–1131. doi:10.1093/ije/dyn086

Meteorological Development Bureau (2010) Daily weather data. Thai Meteorological Department, Ministry of Information and Communication Technology, Bangkok

National Statistical Office (2008) The population and housing census. Ministry of Information and Communication Technology, Thailand. http://service.nso.go.th/nso/thailand/dataFile/04/J04W/J04W/th/0.htm. Accessed 22 May 2009

O'Neill MS, Hajat S, Zanobetti A, Ramirez-Aguilar M, Schwartz J (2005) Impact of control for air pollution and respiratory epidemics on the estimated associations of temperature and daily mortality. Int J Biometeorol 50(2):121–129. doi:10.1007/s00484-005-0269-z

Pan WH, Li LA, Tsai MJ (1995) Temperature extremes and mortality from coronary heart disease and cerebral infarction in elderly Chinese. Lancet 345:353–355. doi:10.1016/S0140-6736(95)90341-0

Patz JA, Campbell-Lendrum D, Holloway T, Foley JA (2005) Impact of regional climate change on human health. Nature 438(7066):310–317. doi:10.1038/nature04188

Pudpong N, Hajat S (2011) High temperature effects on out-patient visits and hospital admissions in Chiang Mai, Thailand. Sci Total Environ 409:5260–5267. doi:10.1016/j.scitotenv.2011.09.005

Royston P, Sauerbrei W (2008) Multivariable model-building: A pragmatic approach to regression analysis based on fractional polynomials for modelling continuous variables. Wiley Series in Probability and Statistics. John Wiley & Sons, Ltd England

Saez M, Sunyer J, Castellsague J, Murillo C, Anto JM (1995) Relationship between weather temperature and mortality: a time series analysis approach in Barcelona. Int J Epidemiol 24(3):576–582

Stafoggia M, Forastiere F, Agostini D, Biggeri A, Bisanti L, Cadum E, Caranci N, De'Donato F, De Lisio S, De Maria M, Michelozzi P, Miglio R, Pandolfi P, Picciotto S, Rognoni M, Russo A, Scarnato C, Perucci CA (2006) Vulnerability to heat-related mortality: multicity, population-based, case-crossover analysis. Epidemiology 17(3):315–323. doi:10.1097/01.ede.0000208477.36665.34

Stafoggia M, Forastiere F, Michelozzi P, Perucci CA (2009) Summer temperature-related mortality. Epidemiology 20(4):575–583. doi:10.1097/EDE.0b013e31819ecdf0

Stata (2011) Stata 12. Stata Corporation, TX

Steadman RG (1979) The assessment of sultriness. Part I: A temperature-humidity index based on human physiology and clothing science. Appl Meteorol 18(7):861–873

Taniguchi M (2006) Anthropogenic effects on subsurface temperature in Bangkok. Clim Past Discuss 2:831–846

Tawatsupa B, Lim LL-Y, Kjellstrom T, Seubsman S, Sleigh A, the Thai Cohort Study team (2010) The association between overall health, psychological distress, and occupational heat stress among a large national cohort of 40,913 Thai workers. Global Health Action 3:5034. doi:10.3402/gha.v3i0.5034

Tawatsupa B, Lim LL-Y, Kjellstrom T, Seubsman S, Sleigh A, the Thai Cohort Study team (2012) Association between occupational heat stress and kidney disease among 37,816 workers in the Thai Cohort Study (TCS). J Epidemiol 22(3):251–260. doi:10.2188/jea.JE20110082

Thai Meteorological Department (2009) Future climate change projection in Thailand. Meteorological Department, Thailand

Tong S, Wang XY, Barnett AG (2010) Assessment of heat-related health impacts in Brisbane, Australia: comparison of different heatwave definitions. PLoS One 5(8):e12155. doi:10.1371/journal.pone.0012155

The association between temperature and mortality in tropical middle income Thailand from 1999 to 2008

Electronic supplementary material

- **Supplementary Material 1:** Formulas for calculation of age-sex adjusted death rates (ADR), Wet Bulb Globe Temperature (WBGT), and Heat Index (HI)

- **Supplementary Material 2:** Main features of sequential regression models developed to relate adjusted death rates and weather condition in Thailand, 1999 to 2008

- **Supplementary Material 3:** National monthly summary statistics for mean, minimum, and maximum province levels for adjusted death rates and weather measurements (N=5,599)

- **Supplementary Material 4:** Mean regional values across 10 years by 4 regions in Thailand (N=5,599 province-months)

- **Supplementary Material 5:** Monthly average values of weather and air pollution by regions (N=1,025 province-months)

Supplementary Material 1: Formulas for calculation of age-sex adjusted death rates (ADR), Wet Bulb Globe Temperature (WBGT), and Heat Index (HI)

1) Calculation of Age-sex adjusted death rates (per 100,000 population)

Daily death counts by age group and sex (d_{ikm}) were then summed into monthly death counts by age group and sex (D_{ikm}) for month m of province k. Then D_{ikm} were calculated as monthly age-sex specific death rates (SDR_{ikm} per 100,000 population). Within each year, the SDR_{ikm} for each of the 18 age-sex groups were multiplied with the standard weights for that group derived from the standard Thai population for that year (w_i), and summed across the relevant age group and sex to get monthly age-sex adjusted death rates for that month in each of the 10 years (ADR_{km} per 100,000 population).

$$ADR_{km} \text{ (per 100,000 population)} \quad = \quad \sum_i w_i \, SDR_{ikm} \qquad (1)$$

When; SDR_{ikm} = Age-sex specific death rate (per 100,000 persons) in month m and province k;

$SDR_{ikm} = D_{ikm} / p_{ik}$

D_{ikm} = Number of deaths by age and sex in month m and province k

p_{ik} = Mid-year population by age and sex in province k

w_i = Standard weights representing the relative age and sex distribution of the standard population; $w_i = P_i / \sum_i P_i$

P_i = Population by age and sex in the standard population; $P_i = \sum_k p_{ik}$

i = 1, 2, 3, ..., 18 age-sex groups (9 age groups and 2 sexes)

2) Calculation of Wet Bulb Globe Temperature (WBGT) (Gagge AP and Nishi Y 1976)

WBGT = 0.567 * Tmax + 0.216*(Humid/100 * 6.105 * exp (17.27 * Tmax/(237.7 + Tmax))) + 3.38

When; Tmax = Maximum Temperature ($^\circ$C)

Humid = Relative Humidity (%)

3) Calculation of Heat Index (HI) (Steadman 1979)

HI = (-42.379 + ((2.04901523 * (Tmax * 9 / 5 + 32)) + (10.1433127 * Humid) - (0.22475541 * (Tmax * 9 / 5 + 32) * Humid) - (6.83783 * 10 ^ -3 * (Tmax * 9 / 5 + 32) ^ 2) - (5.481717 * 10 ^ -2 * Humid ^ 2) + (1.22874 * 10 ^ -3 * (Tmax * 9 / 5 + 32) ^ 2 * Humid) + (8.5282 * 10 ^ -4 * (Tmax * 9 / 5 + 32) * Humid ^ 2) - (1.99 * 10 ^ -6 * (Tmax * 9 / 5 + 32) ^ 2 * Humid ^ 2)) - 32) / 9 * 5

When; Tmax = Maximum Temperature ($^\circ$C)

Humid = Relative Humidity (%)

Supplementary Material 2: Main features of sequential regression models developed to relate adjusted death rates and weather condition in Thailand, 1999 to 2008

Model	Details	Independent variables	Fitted models and outputs
A	MFP model with stepwise selection ($p<0.001$) for significant weather variables for overall Thailand	3 main weather variables (the 3 other weather variables not $p<0.001$)	One fitted model using functional (transformed) forms of the 3 significant variables ($p<0.001$) for overall Thailand (1 model)
B	MFP model with stepwise selection (0.001) for overall Thailand (1 model)	6 main weather variables [a] and 15 interactions of main variables	20 fitted models of - overall Thailand (1 model) - regions (4 models) - seasons (3 models) - season*region (12 models) All models use the same functional (trans) forms of weather variables and significant interactions
C	7 MFP models with stepwise selection at 0.001 - region (4 models) - season (3 models)	6 main weather variables [a] and 15 interactions of main variables	All functional forms of variables and significant interactions from MFP selection of any region or any season use to fit 20 models of overall Thailand (1 model) by regions (4 models) by seasons (3 models) by season*region (12 models)
D	- Multivariable linear regression (models D1 – D3) - MFP (model D4)	Model includes combination of 2 functional forms of maximum temperature ($Tmax_1$ and $Tmax_2$) and $Tmax_1$ by region $Tmax_1$ by season $Tmax_2$ by region $Tmax_2$ by season	Each model in the set of model D produced 12 region-season-specific coefficients for transformed maximum temperature – first by maximum temperature only, then with other untransformed weather variables, then with weather variable interactions, then with all weather variables transformed (4 models)
E	- Multivariable linear regression (models E1, E2, E3, E5) - MFP (model E4)	2 functional forms of Tmax combined -$Tmax_1$ by region*season -$Tmax_2$ by region*season	Model E set is same as model D plus interactions of region-season (5 models)

[a] The 6 weather variables are mean temperature, maximum temperature, minimum temperature, wind speed, precipitation, and dew point temperature

Supplementary Material 3: National monthly summary statistics for mean, minimum, and maximum province levels for adjusted death rates and weather measurements (N=5,599)

No.	Detail of variables	Mean	Std. Dev.	Min	Max
	Age-sex adjusted death rates (ADR)[a]	50.3	8.8	23.8	91.5
1	Mean temperature (°C)	27.4	2.1	17.4	32.7
2	Maximum temperature (°C)	32.7	2.0	24.3	40.0
3	Minimum temperature (°C)	22.5	2.8	10.6	30.5
4	Average dew point temperature (°C)	21.9	2.9	10.6	26.5
5	Average precipitation in 24hrs (mm.)	2.2	2.8	0.0	25.4
6	Maximum wind speed (m/s)	9.2	2.9	1.8	23.4

[a] ADR = National monthly average of monthly age-sex adjusted provincial death rates

Supplementary Material 4: Mean regional values across 10 years by 4 regions in Thailand (N=5,599 province-months)

Average values by regions	North	Northeast	Centre	South
Age-sex adjusted death rates (ADR) [a]	53.9	49.4	51.2	46.1
Monthly mean temperature (°C)	26.8	27.1	28.3	27.8
Monthly maximum temperature (°C)	32.7	32.6	33.4	32.2
Monthly minimum temperature (°C)	21.3	22.1	23.8	23.7
Monthly average dew point temperature (°C)	20.9	21.1	22.6	23.5
Monthly average precipitation in 24hrs (mm.) [b]	0.8	0.7	0.9	1.1
Monthly average maximum wind speed (m/s) [b]	2.1	2.3	2.3	2.5
Total N = 5,599 province-months	1,644	1,668	970	1,317

[a] ADR = Regional monthly average of monthly age-sex adjusted provincial death rates

[b] Values of precipitation and wind speed are in log transforms "ln(x+1)"

Supplementary Material 5: Monthly average values of weather and air pollution by regions (N=1,025 province-months)

Average values by regions	North	Northeast	Centre	South	Overall
Age-sex adjusted death rates (ADR)	60.8	52.4	53.5	51.8	54.5
Monthly mean temperature (°C)	26.5	27.2	28.5	27.9	27.6
Monthly maximum temperature (°C)	32.7	32.6	33.2	32.3	32.7
Monthly minimum temperature (°C)	20.8	22.2	24.4	24.0	23.0
Monthly average dew point temperature (°C)	19.9	21.2	22.8	23.6	22.0
Monthly average precipitation in 24hrs (mm.) [a]	0.7	0.9	0.8	1.4	1.0
Monthly average maximum wind speed (m/s) [a]	2.4	2.4	2.4	2.5	2.4
Monthly mean SO_2 concentration (ppb) [a]	0.7	1.1	1.3	0.9	1.0
Monthly mean NO_2 concentration (ppb) [a]	2.0	2.7	2.6	2.1	2.3
Monthly mean O_3 concentration (ppb) [a]	2.7	2.9	2.9	2.4	2.7
Monthly mean CO concentration (ppm) [a]	0.4	0.6	0.5	0.4	0.5
Monthly mean PM_{10} concentration ($\mu g/m^3$) [a]	3.8	3.7	3.9	3.6	3.8
Monthly maximum SO_2 concentration (ppb) [a]	1.6	1.6	2.2	1.3	1.7
Monthly maximum NO_2 concentration (ppb) [a]	3.0	3.1	3.3	2.6	3.0
Monthly maximum O_3 concentration (ppb) [a]	3.4	3.3	3.6	3.0	3.3
Monthly maximum CO concentration (ppm) [a]	0.9	0.8	0.9	0.6	0.8
Monthly maximum PM_{10} concentration ($\mu g/m^3$) [a]	4.6	4.2	4.5	4.1	4.4

[a] Values of precipitation, wind speed and all air pollution are in log transforms "ln(x+1)"

CHAPTER 8: DISCUSSION AND CONCLUSION

8.1 Overview

The findings of this thesis confirm that there is a multi-faceted association between heat stress and adverse health outcomes in a tropical developing country, Thailand. Some groups of the Thai working population are at high risk of heat stress effects, especially males in physical jobs. These worker effects included psychological distress, workplace injuries, and kidney disease. Also, the general Thai population is at risk of heat stress effects on overall health, energy levels, daily activities, life satisfaction, and personal well-being. The above findings raise considerable concern about the prevalent population effects of heat stress in Thailand. Of even more concern is the finding linking temperature and mortality across the country. Moreover, heat-related deaths are expected to increase in the future as a result of climate change and warming in Thailand.

In this thesis, the previous results sections (Chapters 3-7) present the significant findings regarding the health impacts of heat stress. Each of these results chapters has its own discussion section. This final chapter presents overall key findings as well as the strengths and limitations of this thesis. It concludes by drawing attention to future research directions for health impact assessment from climate change, the significance of this thesis, and implications for public health in Thailand.

8.2 Key findings

The five studies reported in Chapters 3-7 address the three research questions of this thesis (see section 1.4 in Chapter 1).

The first research question is "Are there any health impacts from heat stress in Thai workers?". This thesis provides evidence for strong and significant associations between heat stress at work in tropical Thailand and poor overall health, psychological distress, occupational injury, and incident kidney disease (Tawatsupa et al. 2010; Tawatsupa et al. 2012b; Tawatsupa et al. 2013). Low socioeconomic status and physical job type are related factors that can increase the heat stress effects. The most vulnerable group to heat stress effects on health is the male workers in physical jobs.

The second research question is "Are there any health impacts of heat stress on the overall Thai population?". The thesis demonstrates that heat stress not only affects the health of workers but also has an impact on the overall population. Climate-related heat stress in tropical Thailand is associated with health and well-being when the heat interferes with daily activities such as sleep, housework, travel, and exercise. This problem of heat interference affected up to one fifth of the study cohort. These findings add to the limited literature on the heat stress effects in the Thai population (Tawatsupa et al. 2012c).

In addition to the above effects on work and daily activities the thesis revealed that there is a strong national relationship between maximum temperature and mortality in Thailand (Tawatsupa et al. 2012a). Maximum temperature is a useful indicator of heat exposure in health risk assessment. Overall, the association with mortality is U-shaped and 33°C is the minimum-mortality temperature in Thailand. The non-linear temperature-mortality patterns found in this thesis for a tropical zone hot and humid climate in Thailand are similar to patterns reported for earlier temperate zone climate studies (Martens 1998; Armstrong 2006). The death rates increase when maximum temperature increase with the highest rates in the North and Central during hot months.

The third research question is "Are these health impacts expected to increase due to climate change and the projected increase of temperature?". Over the last century, average temperature in Thailand has already increased, and further increase is expected as a result of climate change. An estimation of the impact of a 4°C increase in temperature, as projected for Thailand by 2100, revealed that overall the net increase in expected mortality by region ranges from 5% to 13% unless preventive measures are adopted (Tawatsupa et al. 2012a). By taking into account the expected future population of Thailand it can be calculated that by 2100 the annual deaths will increase by 32,000 due to the 4°C increase in temperature unless preventive measures are adopted across the nation.

8.3 Strengths of this thesis

The main advantage of the thesis is full access to large national datasets - the Thai Cohort Study (TCS) data and the four national government databases on weather, air pollution, mortality, and population.

The advantage of the first four studies in Chapters 3-6 is access to the TCS data derived from a large national cohort of Thai workers and other Thai adults. It represents working-age Thais reasonably well for geographic location, age, and socioeconomic status for both sexes (Sleigh et al. 2008). Also, the follow-up data allows us to analyse incidence rates and to categorise heat exposure by degree of prolongation.

The cohort data have a wide range of values for variables of interest, revealing the relationship between heat stress and health outcomes. The study group is very large (N=87,134) so the epidemiological results remain substantial and statistically significant even when extensively adjusted for a wide array of potential confounding or explanatory variables. Another strength of the TCS is that the cohort members are better educated than average Thais of the same age and sex. This difference enabled us to gather complex information on heat exposure and health outcomes for large numbers by questionnaire. The TCS questionnaires included many questions on a wide array of exposures and health outcomes. It should be noted that questions on heat stress and health outcomes were in different parts of the questionnaire, so the respondents would not be aware of any connection between the exposures and the outcomes.

The main study is reported in Chapter 7 and shows the association between weather and mortality. One strength of this study is access to the four large national datasets for mortality, population, weather, and air pollution spanning 10 years obtained from various official sources. Weather condition and mortality rates were analysed across Thailand by seasons and regions adjusting for possible confounding by air pollution and its interactions and were quite adequate for monthly averaging, which it is a suitable technique in a stable climate of Thailand. The analysis used advanced statistical methods of Multivariable Fractional Polynomial regression (MFP) which it is suited for continuous variables and non-linear associations by produced optimal transformation of weather and air pollution variables that enable detailed analysis of the temperature-mortality relationship. Furthermore, the final model permits estimates of mortality outcomes if temperatures rise according to the 4°C global warming scenario in Thailand.

8.4 Limitations of this thesis

The main limitation of this thesis is that the cross-sectional studies using TCS data could not directly establish that all those health outcomes arose as a result of heat stress. There are some difficulties in inferring causality between heat stress and health outcomes. Hence there is a need for further study with longitudinal analysis and this is planned for the 8-year follow up in 2013.

Unfortunately, the data did not permit ascertainment of the time relationship of the heat stress exposures and the health outcomes. However, the associations found in this thesis are unlikely to arise by chance ($p < 0.001$) and this fits well with an epidemiological model linking heat stress to increased health risks. Additionally, the heat-related health outcome models are supported by a dose response whereby more frequent heat stress exposure associates with increased odds of worse health outcomes.

Another limitation in this study of occupational heat stress is the unknown source or nature of the heat stress and that the actual work situations were not reported in the cohort data. Indeed, direct measurements of work environments or health outcomes have not been done so the study reported here must be classified as preliminary in nature. Further studies are needed for more detailed direct observations in informative work settings to validate our findings and explore the underlying mechanisms.

Also of concern is the estimation of heat stress effects on mortality in the future as a result of an expected increase in temperature of 4°C. This estimate has some limitations. For example, the estimation of heat-related deaths if temperatures rise in the future needs further study to take into account uncertainties regarding demographic change, effectiveness of the health care system, intensity, duration and frequency of projected climate change, as well as potential adaptation (IPCC 2007).

8.5 Future research

Occupational heat stress requires more public health attention. Further studies are needed to accurately characterise workplace temperature and humidity, air movement, radiant temperature, actual health outcomes, and work performance in various settings in Thailand. This is especially important as the workforce structure changes from informal to formal employment as a result of economic development (Kelly et al. 2010; National Statistical Office 2012).

Now direct observations of heat stress and its effects in informative work settings are needed to add information on water intake, dehydration, physical and biomechanical mechanisms generating heat stress and linking it to medical records or actual health outcomes. As well, there is a need to investigate heat-related ill-health or injury in different regions of Thailand because the geography and heat stress are different. For example, in Thailand temperatures vary considerably during the day and night in the North but little in the South.

This thesis documents the adverse effect of high maximum temperature on the population in Thailand. For each region and season there are different optimum temperatures and temperature-mortality slopes. However, the exact physical mechanisms and at-risk subpopulations are unclear and further investigation is needed to determine who is actually dying and how high maximum temperatures are causing the deaths.

Heat stress effects in different age groups are of particular interest, especially mortality among working age groups (15-64 years) (Kjellstrom et al. 2009a). For most of the year, this group is often exposed to heavy labour outdoors during hot weather (Tawatsupa et al. 2010; Tawatsupa et al. 2012b). Furthermore, heat risks will steadily increase over time because the Thai population is ageing. The elderly are at high risk as their thermoregulations are impaired and many of them have less protective measures to avoid heat stress (Diaz et al. 2002; Basu et al. 2005; Hajat et al. 2007).

Furthermore, future research of heat stress and mortality relationship should use fine-grained individual data instead of large-scale data of overall Thailand. We can select the weather stations on the completeness of measurements and representation of population exposure. The sampling procedure should select people whose home locations are close to the nearest available weather station (eg. within 10 kilometres radius from weather station located). The weather values recorded by the nearest weather station can be considered more representative of heat stress exposure for those populations who live nearby than the populations who live far from that station. However, we need the information of individual data on home address and weather stations' location to conduct this analysis.

8.6 Significance of this thesis

Previous studies have shown that heat stress is an important risk factor for health and well-being (Basu and Samet 2002a; Hajat et al. 2006; Kovats and Hajat 2008; McMichael et al. 2008; Kjellstrom 2009b; Hajat and Kosatky 2010). This thesis is one of the first large scale studies providing evidence for an association between heat stress and adverse health outcomes in Thailand. These findings are particularly important at present because the existing heat stress problem will worsen if global warming continues and tropical Thailand become even more thermally stressful. Thai population will be exposed to excessive heat in hot and humid environment. If they cannot adapt to heat stress, they can experience severe psychological distress or develop long term conditions such as chronic depression or chronic anxiety disorders (Hansen et al. 2008a).

Furthermore, heat stress diminished mental ability and increased injury risks (Ramsey 1995), and others have noted increased suicide risk (Anderson 2001; Page et al. 2007; Berry et al. 2010). These findings support the study reported by Kjellstrom et al (2009a) that heat stress can increases the risk of ill-health and serious injury, especially among workers who are exposed to hot and humid work environments in low income-tropical countries (Kjellstrom et al. 2009b). The combination of hot weather and high humidity together with physical exertion and dehydration can cause potentially heat-related illness or heat exhaustion which could increase injury and associated costs as well as reduce physical performance and productivity. Furthermore, a rapid increase in kidney disease is already occurring in tropical Thailand. Heat stress should be regarded as a possible cause, in which case global warming will increase the risk.

In Thailand, an anticipated increase in temperature from climate changes, as well as the ageing and growing urban population, could significantly increase existing heat stress impacts on health and well-being. The results show the largest effects of maximum temperature on mortality were in the inland tropical zones of Thailand. Unless the population is protected, global warming will increase the number of hot-deaths and decrease the cold-deaths in the Thai population. This will be especially prominent in urban areas due to heat island effect. If global warming extends to an increase of 4°C (Thai Meteorological Department 2009), our findings suggest that death rates will increase substantially especially in the hot and wet months of tropical inland zones, and this will affect much of Thailand.

8.7 Implications for public health

The heat stress effects detected in this study translate to a significant public health burden of preventable heat-related health outcomes among Thai workers and overall Thai population.

8.7.1 Health impacts from heat stress in Thai workers

Thai workers must take safety precautions while working under heat stress and policymakers should develop the occupational health and safety interventions to prevent heat-related illness and occupational injury which is urgently needed given the looming threat of global warming.

More attention is needed to the health of tropical workers, especially male workers doing physical jobs during hot weather or under prolonged heat stress. Maintaining hydration must be emphasised for physical workers in Thailand, and this requires a health-behaviour intervention. In addition, the improvement in urban infrastructure and also construction of buildings for workplaces must account for indoor climate while minimising the use of energy-consuming air conditioning systems. Also, prevention of heat stress-related health outcomes through education, training and procedures is needed to protect workers in all types of work environments.

8.7.2 Health impacts from heat stress in Thai population

The associations between heat stress and well-being outcomes as well as mortality among Thai population reported here is a great concern. There is a need to improve public health programs (such as prevention, health care and early warning systems) and increase public awareness regarding the risks of heat stress in daily life which are higher in such a tropical environment.

The health risk from heat stress will steadily increase over time because the Thai population is ageing. The elderly are at high risk as their thermoregulations are impaired and many of them have less protective measures to avoid heat stress (Diaz et al. 2002; Basu et al. 2005; Hajat et al. 2007). In this thesis, maximum temperature can be used as an indicator for heat stress exposure of the population in Thailand. So, maximum temperature monitoring would help public health surveillance of this risk.

Overall, the results of this thesis are useful for health impact assessment for the present situation and the public health implications of climate change for tropical

Thailand. The present health impacts of heat stress would be expected to increase with global warming. Rising temperatures in the future along with the rapidly growing urban populations in tropical and developing countries may worsen the health outcomes.

APPENDIX

Appendix A: Additional details of the national data

Introduction

The study on the association between weather and mortality in Thailand highlights the health effects of heat stress during the early 21st century. This study used data from four national datasets including weather, air pollution, mortality and population data from 1999 to 2008 (Figure A1).

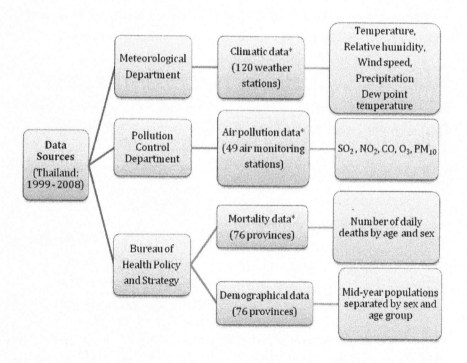

*This data are available and represent daily observations from 1999 to 2008

Figure A1 Data source for study effects of heat stress on mortality in Thailand

This section describes the source of the four datasets and issues to be considered in relation to measurements and validity of weather, air pollution, mortality and population data.

1. Weather data

Weather data are very important for investigating the relationship between heat stress and mortality. The weather data are routinely collected from local weather stations. All weather data are recorded and sent to the Thai Meteorological Department (TMD) (Meteorological Development Bureau 2010). TMD is the centre for processing and collecting data from a total of 120 local weather stations in Thailand. All stations are fixed-site stations which measure the weather data by following the international procedures of the World Meteorological Organization (WMO) (Meteorological Development Bureau 2010). For data quality control, all equipment at the weather stations are checked and calibrated for the accuracy of measurements annually.

For this study, the daily weather data from 1 January 1999 to 31 December 2008 were obtained from TMD. Additionally, five weather stations were selected for site visits in order to investigate the data recording and reporting system. The selected weather stations were;

1) Northern Meteorological Center in Chiang Mai
2) Chiang Mai weather station
3) Ayuttaya agrometeorological station
4) Pathumthani weather station
5) Bang Na weather station

All meteorological weather stations have meteorological fields where the meteorological instruments are located and operated for measuring all weather conditions (Figure A2). The meteorological field is an outdoor field approximately 20 x 30 feet and distant from any trees and buildings.

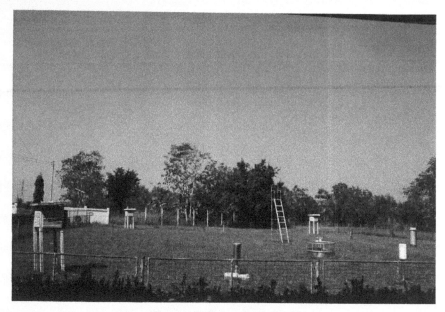

Figure A2 Meteorological field

Each meteorological weather station has at least one technical officer who is in charge of measuring and collecting the weather data every day. They are responsible for monitoring and reporting extreme weather events in the area where the weather station is located. They also report all weather data to TMD central database by following the international code of practice of WMO. The weather measurements at the local weather stations can be separated into two groups;

1) *Required weather measurements*; all local weather stations need to report some basic weather variables to the TMD central database. Those basic weather variables include mean, minimum, and maximum temperature, relative humidity, precipitation, air pressure and wind speed.

2) *Additional weather measurements;* some local weather stations can measure additional meteorological conditions because relevant equipment is available. (eg thermograph, hygrograph, sunshine length measurements, evaporation measurements)

This section describes measurement methods for each weather variable in the dataset that we obtained from TMD. The weather variables include mean, maximum and minimum temperature (°C), relative humidity (%), rain during 24 hours (mm), wind speed in 24 hours (m/s) and dew point temperature (°C).

1.1) Daily maximum and minimum temperature

Air temperature is the main variable used in describing the effects of heat stress. Generally, air temperature can be measured by using thermometer or data logger which are available at all local weather stations.

Daily maximum temperature (Tmax) is the highest temperature and daily minimum temperature (Tmin) is the lowest temperature (in °C) measured within the 24 hours. Tmax is observed between 7pm (local time) of the day before to 7 pm of the current day. Tmin is observed between 7am of the day before to 7am of the current day. These temperature observations correspond to the daily temperature cycle. In other words, the early morning Tmin usually follows the afternoon Tmax in that day.

Tmax and Tmin are measured by the thermometer in the thermometer screen (Figure A3 and A4), a two-shelf cabinet with white colour for preventing heat from sun radiation. The door of the thermometer screen always directs to the North or the South direction. The cabinet is located 1.25 to 2.00 meters above ground level or around eye level.

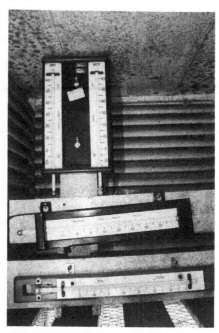

Figure A3 Dry-wet bulbs psychrometer, maximum, and minimum thermometer

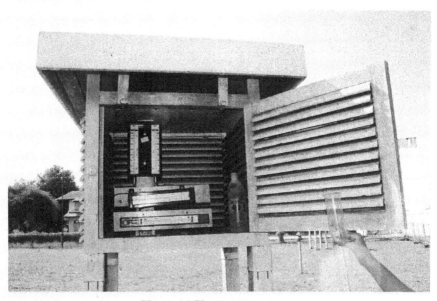

Figure A4 Thermometer screen

1.2) Relative humidity

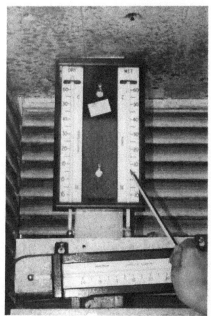

Figure A5 Dry-wet bulb psychrometer

During hot conditions, water is heated and evaporates to the surrounding environment; the resulting amount of water in the air will provide humidity. In meteorology, air humidity can be expressed by vapour pressure, dew point temperature and relative humidity.

Relative humidity (in %) is the ratio between the actual amount of water vapour in the air and the maximum amount of water vapour that the air can hold at that air temperature (Bureau of Meteorology 2011). Hence, the relative humidity varies during the day depending on air temperature. Dewpoint temperature (in °C), is more stable than relative humidity as it is the temperature that the air needs to be cooled to make the air saturated.

Relative humidity is usually measured by using the psychrometer which is set up in the thermometer screen. The psychrometer measures two values of temperatures from dry- and wet-bulb thermometers (Figure A5). The dry-bulb thermometer commonly measures air temperature and the wet-bulb thermometer measures temperature from a thermometer which is covered with saturated cloths in the basement. The difference between the dry and wet bulb temperatures is called the wet-bulb depression, and this value can be calculated to get the relative humidity and dew point temperature. The air temperature and relative humidity are measured every three hours which start measuring at 1am, 4am, 7am, 10am, 1pm, 4pm, 7pm and 10pm every day. Then, all the measuring records within a day are used to calculate daily mean temperature and daily mean relative humidity.

1.3) Precipitation

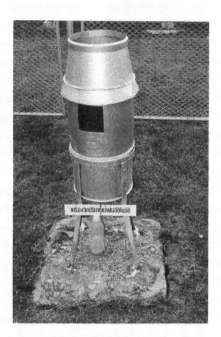 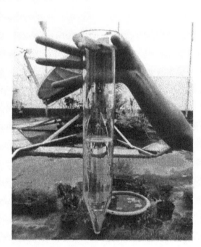

Figure A6 Rain gauge

Rain gauges are used for measuring precipitation (Figure A6). The gauge is set on plain ground with the height not over one meter from the ground and without any barriers around. The rain gauge has a diameter of eight inches that can catch rain water into the cylinder at the bottom. The daily rain level can be measured in millimetres by reading the gauge.

1.4) Wind speed

Wind speed and wind direction are measured using the wind that moves toward the station at 11 metres high from the ground. Wind direction is observed by the wind vanes (Figure A7). An anemometer is used for measuring wind speed which is reported in knots, the international unit.

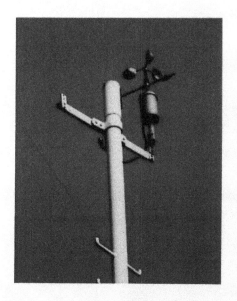

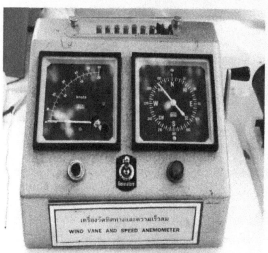

Figure A7 Cup and wind vanes (top) and anemometer (bottom)

1.5) Data Logger (automatic weather system)

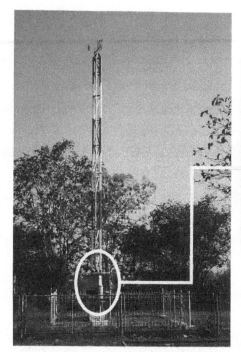
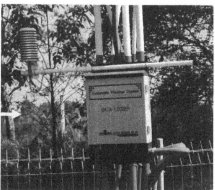

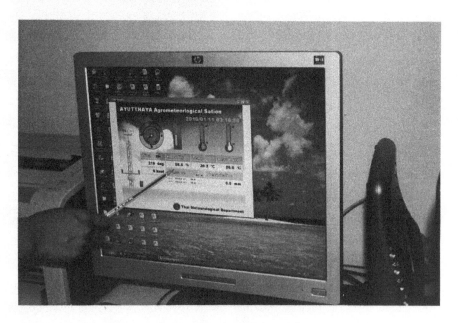

Figure A8 Data logger (automatic weather system)

All local weather stations follow the international standard of WMO for measuring and recording all weather data. There are two types of data recording systems; the self-recording system by staff every three hours of every day, and the automatic-recording system by data logger (Figure A8).

The data logger is a machine that each minute automatically records the real-time data digitally. All weather data from the data logger is sent to the TMD central database via an online system. It can measure all basic weather variables including temperature, relative humidity, dew point temperature, rain, wind direction, wind speed and solar radiation. The technical officer at weather stations can check the accuracy and validity of weather data by comparing the data recorded from these two systems.

2) Air quality data

Due to concerns regarding the interactive effects of temperature and air pollution on mortality, ambient air quality data were derived from the Pollution Control Department (PCD), Ministry of Natural Resource and Environment, Thailand. The Air Quality and Noise Management Bureau, PCD is responsible for controlling an air quality monitoring network system and monitoring ambient air quality in Thailand under the Enhancement and Conservation of National Environment Quality Act of 1992.

The air quality monitoring network system at PCD consists of two parts: the central air quality monitoring system and air quality monitoring stations. The central monitoring system at PCD is a central automatic system which obtains data that is reported continuously on-line and in real-time from air quality monitoring stations. The central monitoring system can collect data from 51 local air quality monitoring stations, which are located in 25 provinces across the country. The local air monitoring stations are located in urban areas at least 50 meters distant from a main road. Due to air pollution problems from traffic in Bangkok, there are seven mobile stations that are located on the road sites. These mobile stations are located less than 10 meters away from main roads.

The air monitoring stations measure level of carbon monoxide (CO), nitrogen dioxide (NO_2), sulphur dioxide (SO_2), ozone (O_3), and particulate matter with diameter less than 10 microns (PM_{10}), as well as weather data (wind speed, wind direction, temperature, solar radiation, atmospheric pressure, rainfall, and noise). Each local air-monitoring station automatically reports all real-time data to the central air quality monitoring system every hour continuously. Then, the central processing system at PCD is responsible for validating and analysing data daily according to quality assurance procedures by the Air Quality and Noise Management Bureau. Air pollution data are reported and updated on the PCD website at 9am everyday for monitoring purposes and for open access by the public. The measurement methods of air pollution are described in Table A1.

Table A1 Air pollution measurements by the air monitoring stations in Thailand

Pollutants	Measurement Method	Average period	Standard of maximum concentration
Carbon Monoxide (CO) (in ppm)	Non-dispersive infrared detection	1 hour	No more than 30 ppm
Nitrogen Dioxide (NO_2) (in ppb)	Chemiluminescence	1 hour	No more than 170 ppb
Sulphur Dioxide (SO_2) (in ppb)	Ultraviolet fluorescence	1 hour	No more than 300 ppb
Ozone (O_3) (in ppb)	Ultraviolet absorption photometry	1 hour	No more than 100 ppb
Particular Matter with diameter less than 10 microns (PM_{10}) (in ug/m^3)	Gravimetric/Beta Ray absorption	24 hour	No more than 120 ug/m^3

Source: Air Quality and Noise Management Bureau, 2009

In this study, the air pollution dataset between 1999 and 2008 were derived from the central air quality automatic monitoring system at PCD consisting of air pollution concentrations based on daily average values (10am yesterday to 9am today). These air pollution data are reported from 49 air quality monitoring stations; 15 stations in Bangkok and 34 stations in 22 other provinces between 1 January 1999 and 31 December 2008. All air pollution data reflect the general background urban air pollution level which included 1-hour CO, 1-hour NO_2, 1-hour SO_2, 1-hour O_3 and 24-hours PM_{10}.

3) Mortality data

Mortality has always been a key health endpoint in epidemiological studies. It is a well defined health outcome and widely used in studies of the effect of heat stress or weather variations. In Thailand, there are well-established systems of civil registration including compulsory death registration (Health Information System Development Office 2010). The death registration in Thailand started with a manual collecting system since 1837 and it was converted to a computerised recording system in 1996.

For individual death registration, notification of death has to be done by the deceased's family within 24 hours after death or after the dead body has been found. Then they obtain doctor's death notification form from hospitals or local public health offices which is necessary for funeral purposes and for formally registering the dead person at the civil registration office in the locality where the death occurred. After the official recording of deaths, the local civil registration office issues two copies of the civil death certificate; one copy of the civil death certificate is issued to the person who notifies for the funeral, while another copy is retained in the system. The copy of the civil death certificate in the system is electronically sent to the central database of civil registration at Bureau of Registration and Administration, Department of Local Administration at the Ministry of Interior (MOI) for updating and stopping the decedent's household registration. A copy is also sent to the mortality databases at the Bureau of Health Policy and Planning at the Ministry of Public Health (MOPH).

Data of the deceased person including name and citizen identification number are removed from the household unit in the civil registration lists. These essential registered mortality statistics are then processed and compiled and are used for producing various key statistics such as death rates, infant deaths, neonatal deaths, or maternal deaths. These statistics are reported and included in the annual reports of public health statistics. These mortality and cause of death data in particular are used to monitor the health status of the Thai population and can be a critical input to public health planning and policy making (Economic and social commission for Asia and the Pacific 2008).

In this study, the daily mortality data for all 76 provinces of Thailand from 1 January 1999 to 31 December 2008 (Bureau of Policy and Strategy 2010a) were obtained in electronic format from the centralised database of death certificates recorded at the Bureau of Health Policy and Planning, MOPH, Thailand. All mortality data covering the country as a whole included age at death (years), sex, date of death, month and year of death, the address of usual residence at time of death by province and underlying causes of death. Causes of death are coded by using ICD-10 (World Health Organization 1993)

4) Mid-year population data

The mid-year national population from 1999 to 2008 were obtained from the MOPH and are linked to the central database at the Bureau of Registration and Administration, MOI. The population data are based on the Thai population at the end of each year derived from the civil registration system at the MOI. For public health reporting the MOPH calculates the annual population figure from the size of the population in the middle of each year; for example calculating mortality rate and producing the annual report of Thailand health profile. These mid-year population data are recorded by province, sex, and age group.

In this study, midyear population figures were categorised by age group: 0-4 years, 5-14 years, 15-24 years, 25-34 years, 35-44 years, 45-54 years, 55-64 years, 65-74 years, and 75 years or over. Age group specific populations were summed to get the total population of Thailand by year from 1999 to 2008 (Bureau of Policy and Strategy 2010b) and validated by comparing with the published statistics of the MOPH or other statistical reports by MOI. Thai population figures were also compared with the population census survey reports from the National Statistical Office (NSO) (National Economic and Social Development Board 2007). The National Statistical Office (NSO) is responsible for carrying out a population census every 10 years. The last census was taken in 2004. This snapshot of the population data is used to check the accuracy of population registration at MOI and MOPH.

REFERENCES

ACGIH (2008) 2008 TLVs and BEIs: Threshold limit values for chemical substances and physical agents and biological exposure indices. American Conference of Governmental Industrial Hygienists, Cincinnati, Ohio

Air Quality and Noise Management Bureau (2010) Daily air quality data. Pollution Control Department, Ministry of National Resources and Environment, Bangkok, Thailand

Akhtar R (2007) Climate change and health and heat wave mortality in India. *Global Environmental Research* 11 (1):51-57.

Anderson BG, Bell ML (2009) Weather-related mortality: How heat, cold, and heat waves affect mortality in the United States. *Epidemiology* 20 (2):205-213.

Anderson C (2001) Heat and violence. *Current Directions in Psychological Science* 10 (1):33-38.

Anderson C, Anderson K, Dorr N, DeNeve K, Flanagan M (2000) Temperature and aggression. *Advances in Experimental Social Psychology* 32:63-133.

Armstrong B (2006) Models for the relationship between ambient temperature and daily mortality. *Epidemiology* 17 (6):624-631.

Armstrong BG, Chalabi Z, Fenn B, Hajat S, Kovats S, Milojevic A, Wilkinson P (2011) Association of mortality with high temperatures in a temperate climate: England and Wales. *Journal of Epidemiology and Community Health* 65 (4):340-345.

Atsamon L, Sangchan L, Thavivongse S Assessment of extreme weather events along the coastal areas of Thailand. In: Eighth Conference on Coastal Atmospheric and Oceanic Prediction and Processes, The 89th American Meteorological Society Annual Meeting, Phoenix, AZ, 2007.

Austin H, Flanders WD, Rothman KJ (1989) Bias arising in case-control studies from selection of controls from overlapping groups. *International Journal of Epidemiology* 18 (3):713-716.

Ayyappan R, Sankar S, Rajkumar P, Balakrishnan K (2009) Work-related heat stress concerns in automotive industries: A case study from Chennai, India. *Global Health Action* 2.

Baccini M, Biggeri A, Accetta G, Kosatsky T, Katsouyanni K, Analitis A, Anderson HR, Bisanti L, D'Ippoliti D, Danova J, Forsberg B, Medina S, Paldy A, Rabczenko D, Schindler C, Michelozzi P (2008) Heat effects on mortality in 15 European cities. *Epidemiology* 19 (5):711-719.

Baccini M, Kosatsky T, Analitis A, Anderson HR, D'Ovidio M, Menne B, Michelozzi P, Biggeri A (2011) Impact of heat on mortality in 15 European cities: attributable deaths under different weather scenarios. *Journal of Epidemiology and Community Health* 65 (1):64-70.

Ballester F, Corella D, Perez-Hoyos S, Saez M, Hervas A (1997) Mortality as a function of temperature. A study in Valencia, Spain, 1991-1993. *International Journal of Epidemiology* 26 (3):551-561.

Bambrick H, Dear K, Woodruff R, Hanigan I, McMichael A (2008) Garnaut climate change review - The impacts of climate change on three health outcomes: Temperature-related mortality and hospitalisations, salmonellosis and other bacterial gastroenteritis, and population at risk from dengue. Cambridge University Press

Bark N (1998) Deaths of psychiatric patients during heat waves. *Psychiatric Services* 49 (8):1088-1090.

Barnett AG (2007) Temperature and cardiovascular deaths in the US elderly: Changes over time. *Epidemiology* 18 (3):369-372.

Baron de Montesquieu (1748) The spirit of laws (trans: Nugent T), vol 1. 1949 edn. The Colonial Press.

Basu R (2009) High ambient temperature and mortality: A review of epidemiologic studies from 2001 to 2008. *Environmental Health* 8 (1):40.

Basu R, Dominici F, Samet JM (2005) Temperature and mortality among the elderly in the United States: a comparison of epidemiologic methods. *Epidemiology* 16 (1):58-66.

Basu R, Malig B (2010) Basu and Malig respond to "Case-crossover methods and preterm birth". *American Journal of Epidemiology* 172 (10):1121-1122.

Basu R, Malig B, Ostro B (2010) High ambient temperature and the risk of preterm delivery. *American Journal of Epidemiology* 172 (10):1108-1117.

Basu R, Samet JM (2002a) An exposure assessment study of ambient heat exposure in an elderly population in Baltimore, Maryland. *Environmental Health Perspective* 110 (12):1219-1224.

Basu R, Samet JM (2002b) Relation between elevated ambient temperature and mortality: A review of the epidemiologic evidence. *Epidemiologic Reviews* 24 (2):190-202.

Bateson TF, Schwartz J (1999) Control for seasonal variation and time trend in case-crossover studies of acute effects of environmental exposures. *Epidemiology* 10 (5):539-544.

Bateson TF, Schwartz J (2001) Selection bias and confounding in case-crossover analyses of environmental time-series data. *Epidemiology* 12 (6):654-661.

Bell ML, O'Neill MS, Ranjit N, Borja-Aburto VH, Cifuentes LA, Gouveia NC (2008) Vulnerability to heat-related mortality in Latin America: A case-crossover study in São Paulo, Brazil, Santiago, Chile and Mexico City, Mexico. *International Journal of Epidemiology* 37 (4):796-804.

Bernard SM, Samet JM, Grambsch A, Ebi KL, Romieu I (2001) The potential impacts of climate variability and change on air pollution-related health effects in the United States. *Environmental Health Perspectives* 109 (2 Suppl):199-209.

Bernard TE, Pourmoghani M (1999) Prediction of workplace wet bulb global temperature. *Applied Occupational and Environmental Hygiene* 14 (2):126-134.

Berry HL, Bowen K, Kjellstrom T (2010) Climate change and mental health: A causal pathways framework. *International Journal of Public Health* 55 (2):123-132.

Blazejczyk K, Epstein Y, Jendritzky G, Staiger H, Tinz B (2012) Comparison of UTCI to selected thermal indices. *International Journal of Biometeorology* 56 (3):515-535.

Bouchama A, Dehbi M, Mohamed G, Matthies F, Shoukri M, Menne B (2007) Prognostic factors in heat wave-related deaths: A meta-analysis. *Archives of Internal Medicine* 167 (20):2170-2176.

Bouchama A, Knochel JP (2002) Heat stroke. *New England Journal of Medicine* 346 (25):1978 - 1988.

Boyd JT (1960) Climate, air pollution, and mortality. *British Journal of Preventive and Social Medicine* 14 (3):123-135.

Braga AL, Zanobetti A, Schwartz J (2001) The time course of weather-related deaths. *Epidemiology* 12 (6):662-667.

Braga AL, Zanobetti A, Schwartz J (2002) The effect of weather on respiratory and cardiovascular deaths in 12 US cities. *Environmental Health Perspectives* 110:859 - 863.

Bridger CA, Ellis FP, Taylor HL (1976) Mortality in St Louis, Missouri, during heat waves in 1936, 1953, 1954, 1955, and 1966. Coroner's cases. *Environmental Research* 12 (1):38-48.

Bridger RS (2003) Introduction to ergonomics. 2nd edition edn. Taylor & Francis, London.

Brikowski TH, Lotan Y, Pearle MS (2008) Climate-related increase in the prevalence of urolithiasis in the United States. *Proceedings of the National Academy of Sciences* 105 (28):9841-9846.

Bull GM, Morton J (1978) Environment, temperature and death rates. *Age and Ageing* 7 (4):210-224.

Bureau of Meteorology (2011) Monitoring the weather. Commonwealth of Australia. http://www.bom.gov.au/info/ftweather/page_18.shtml. Accessed 29 August 2011

Bureau of Policy and Strategy (2010a) Daily mortality data. Office of Permanent Secretary, Ministry of Public Health, Nonthaburi, Thailand

Bureau of Policy and Strategy (2010b) Number of mid-year population. Office of Permanent Secretary, Ministry of Public Health, Nonthaburi, Thailand

Burton, AC (1934) The Application of the Theory of Heat Flow to the study of Energy Metabolism. *Journal of Nutrition*, 7, 497-533.

Campbell-Lendrum D, Corvalan C (2007) Climate change and developing-country cities: implications for environmental health and equity. *Journal of Urban Health* 84 (1 Suppl):i109-117.

Campbell-Lendrum D, Woodruff R (2007) Climate change: Quantifying the health impact at national and local levels. In: Prüss-Üstün A, Corvalán C (eds) WHO Environmental Burden of Disease Series No. 14. World Health Organization, Geneva.

Canadian Centre for Occupational Health and Safety (2008) Hot environments - health effects http://www.ccohs.ca/oshanswers/phys_agents/heat_health.html. Accessed 25 June 2009

Carracedo-Martinez E, Taracido M, Tobias A, Saez M, Figueiras A (2010) Case-crossover analysis of air pollution health effects: A systematic review of methodology and application. *Environmental Health Perspectives* 118 (8):1173-1182.

Cervellin G, Comelli I, Comelli D, Cortellini P, Lippi G, Meschi T, Borghi L (2011) Regional short-term climate variations influence on the number of visits for renal colic in a large urban Emergency Department: Results of a 7-year survey. *Internal and Emergency Medicine* 6 (2):141-147.

Cheung C, Hart M (2012) Climate change and thermal comfort in Hong Kong. *International Journal of Biometeorology*:1-12.

Chidthai-song A (2010) Thailand climate change information. Volume 2: Climate model and future climate. The Thailand Research Fund's Research Development and Co-ordination Center for Global Warming and Climate Change; Thai-GLOB, Bangkok.

Cho KS, Lee SH (1978) Occupational health hazards of mine workers. *Bulletin of the World Health Organization* 56 (2):205-218.

Chung J-Y, Honda Y, Hong Y-C, Pan X-C, Guo Y-L, Kim H (2009) ambient temperature and mortality: An international study in four capital cities of East Asia. *Science of the Total Environment* 408 (2):390-396.

Clarke JF (1972) Some effects of the urban structure on heat mortality. *Environmental Research* 5 (1):93-104.

Confalonieri U, Menne B, Akhtar R, Ebi K, Hauengue M, Kovats RS, Revich B, Woodward A (2007) Human health. Climate change 2007: Impacts, adaptation and vulnerability. Contribution of working group II to the Fourth Assessment Report of the Intergovernmental Panel on Climate Change. ML Parry, OF Canziani, JP Palutikof, PJ van der Linden, CE Hanson. Cambridge University Press, Cambridge, UK, 391-431. http://www.ipcc-wg2.org

Coris EE, Ramirez AM, Van Durme DJ (2004) Heat illness in athletes: the dangerous combination of heat, humidity and exercise. *Sports Medicine* 34 (1):9-16.

Curriero FC, Heiner KS, Samet JM, Zeger SL, Strug L, Patz JA (2002) Temperature and mortality in 11 cities of the Eastern United States. *American Journal of Epidemiology* 155:80-87.

Curriero FC, Samet JM, Zeger SL (2003) Re: "On the use of generalized additive models in time-series studies of air pollution and health" and "Temperature and mortality in 11 cities of the eastern United States". *American Journal of Epidemiology* 158 (1):93-94.

Cusack L, de Crespigny C, Athanasos P (2011) Heatwaves and their impact on people with alcohol, drug and mental health conditions: A discussion paper on clinical practice considerations. *Journal of Advanced Nursing* 67 (4):915-922.

Darrow LA (2010) Invited commentary: Application of case-crossover methods to investigate triggers of preterm birth. *American Journal of Epidemiology* 172 (10):1118-1120.

Dear K, Ranmuthugala G, Kjellström T, Skinner C, Hanigan I (2005) Effects of temperature and ozone on daily mortality during the August 2003 heat wave in France. *Archives of Environmental and Occupational Health* 60 (4):205-212.

Department of Health (2009) Establishment mechanism to responsible for health impacts from climate change in Ministry of Public Health. Department of Health, Ministry of Public Health, Nonthaburi, Thailand.

Dessai S (2003) Heat stress and mortality in Lisbon Part II. An assessment of the potential impacts of climate change. *International Journal of Biometeorology* 48 (1):37-44.

Diaz J, Garcia R, Velazquez de Castro F, Hernandez E, Lopez C, Otero A (2002) Effects of extremely hot days on people older than 65 years in Seville (Spain) from 1986 to 1997. *International Journal of Biometeorology* 46 (3):145-149.

Dominici F (2004) Time-series analysis of air pollution and mortality: A statistical review. *Research Report/Health Effects Institute* (123):3-27; discussion 29-33.

Dominici F, McDermott A, Zeger SL, Samet JM (2002) On the use of generalized additive models in time-series studies of air pollution and health. *American Journal of Epidemiology* 156 (3):193-203.

Donaldson GC, Keatinge WR, Näyhä S (2003) Changes in summer temperature and heat-related mortality since 1971 in North Carolina, South Finland, and Southeast England. *Environmental Research* 91 (1):1-7.

Economic and social commission for Asia and the Pacific (2008) Improving vital statistics and cause of death statistics: The experience of Thailand. Bangkok.

El-Zein A, Tewtel-Salem M (2005) On the association between high temperature and mortality in warm climates. *Science of the Total Environment* 343 (1-3):273-275.

Ellis FP (1972) Mortality from heat illness and heat-aggravated illness in the United States. *Environmental Research* 5 (1):1-58.

Ellis FP (1976) Heat illness. III. Acclimatization. *Transactions of the Royal Society of Tropical Medicine and Hygiene* 70 (5-6):419-425.

Enander AE, Hygge S (1990) Thermal stress and human performance. *Scandinavian Journal of Work, Environment and Health* 16 (1 Suppl):44-50.

Epstein Y, Moran DS (2006) Thermal comfort and the heat stress indices. *Industrial Health* 44 (3):388-398.

Fakheri RJ, Goldfarb DS (2011) Ambient temperature as a contributor to kidney stone formation: Implications of global warming. *Kidney International* 79 (11):1178-1185.

Fiala D, Lomas KJ, Stohrer M (2001) Computer prediction of human thermoregulatory and temperature responses to a wide range of environmental conditions. *International Journal of Biometeorology* 45:143-159.

Fogleman M, Fakhrzadeh L, Bernard TE (2005) The relationship between outdoor thermal conditions and acute injury in an aluminum smelter. *International Journal of Industrial Ergonomics* 35 (1):47-55.

Fouillet A, Rey G, Jougla E, Frayssinet P, Bessemoulin P, Hemon D (2007) A predictive model relating daily fluctuations in summer temperatures and mortality rates. *BMC Public Health* 7:114.

Fouillet A, Rey G, Wagner V, Laaidi K, Empereur-Bissonnet P, Le Tertre A, Frayssinet P, Bessemoulin P, Laurent F, De Crouy-Chanel P, Jougla E, Hemon D (2008) Has the impact of heat waves on mortality changed in France since the European heat wave of summer 2003? A study of the 2006 heat wave. *International Journal of Epidemiology* 37 (2):309-317.

Gagge AP, Nishi Y (1976) Physical indices of the thermal environment. *ASHRAE journal* 18 (47-51).

Gasparrini A, Armstrong B (2010) Time series analysis on the health effects of temperature: advancements and limitations. *Environmental Research* 110 (6):633-638.

Gosling SN, Lowe JA, McGregor GR, Pelling M, Malamud BD (2009a) Associations between elevated atmospheric temperature and human mortality: A critical review of the literature. *Climate Change* 92 (3-4):299-341.

Gosling SN, McGregor GR, Lowe JA (2009b) Climate change and heat-related mortality in six cities Part 2: Climate model evaluation and projected impacts from changes in the mean and variability of temperature with climate change. *International Journal of Biometeorology* 53 (1):31-51.

Gosling SN, McGregor GR, Paldy A (2007) Climate change and heat-related mortality in six cities Part 1: Model construction and validation. *International Journal of Biometeorology* 51 (6):525-540.

Greenberg JH, Bromberg J, Reed CM, Gustafson TL, Beauchamp RA (1983) The epidemiology of heat-related deaths, Texas - 1950, 1970-79, and 1980. *American Journal of Public Health* 73 (7):805-807.

Greenland S (1996) Confounding and exposure trends in case-crossover and case-time-control designs. *Epidemiology* 7 (3):231-239.

Greenland S (2001) Ecologic versus individual-level sources of bias in ecologicestimates of contextual health effects. *International Journal of Epidemiology* 30 (6):1343-1350.

Guest C, Willson K, Woodward A, Hennessy K, Kalkstein L, Skinner C (1999) Climate and mortality in Australia: Retrospective study, 1979-1990, and predicted impacts in five major cities in 2030. *Climate Research* 13:1-15.

Guo Y, Barnett AG, Pan X, Yu W, Tong S (2011) The impact of temperature on mortality in Tianjin, China: A case-crossover design with a distributed lag nonlinear model. *Environmental Health Perspectives* 119 (12):1719-1725.

Guo Y, Punnasiri K, Tong S (2012) Effects of temperature on mortality in Chiang Mai city, Thailand: A time series study. *Environmental Health* 11 (1):36.

Haberman S, Capildeo R, Clifford Rose F (1981) The seasonal variation in mortality from cerebrovascular disease. *Journal of the Neurological Sciences* 52 (1):25-36.

Hajat S, Armstrong B, Baccini M, Biggeri A, Bisanti L, Russo A, Paldy A, Menne B, Kosatsky T (2006) Impact of high temperatures on mortality: Is there an added heat wave effect? *Epidemiology* 17 (6):632-638.

Hajat S, Armstrong BG, Gouveia N, Wilkinson P (2005) Mortality displacement of heat-related deaths: a comparison of Delhi, São Paulo, and London. *Epidemiology* 16 (5):613-620.

Hajat S, Kosatky T (2010) Heat-related mortality: a review and exploration of heterogeneity. *Journal of Epidemiology and Community Health* 64 (9):753-760.

Hajat S, Kovats RS, Lachowycz K (2007) Heat-related and cold-related deaths in England and Wales: who is at risk? *Occupational and Environmental Medicine* 64 (2):93-100.

Hajat S, O'Connor M, Kosatsky T (2010) Health effects of hot weather: From awareness of risk factors to effective health protection. *The Lancet* 375 (9717):856-863.

Hancock PA (1981) Heat stress impairment of mental performance: A revision of tolerance limits. *Aviation Space and Environmental Medicine* 52 (3):177-180.

Hancock PA, Warm JS (1989). A dynamic model of stress and sustained attention. *Human Factors*, 31, 519-537.

Hancock PA, Ross JM, Szalma JL (2007) A meta-analysis of performance response under thermal stressors. *Human Factors: The Journal of the Human Factors and Ergonomics Society* 49 (5):851-877.

Hancock PA, Vasmatzidis I (1998) Human occupational and performance limits under stress: the thermal environment as a prototypical example. *Ergonomics* 41 (8):1169-1191.

Hancock PA, Vasmatzidis I (2003) Effects of heat stress on cognitive performance: The current state of knowledge. *International Journal of Hyperthermia* 19 (3):355-372.

Hansen AL, Bi P, Nitschke M, Ryan P, Pisaniello D, Tucker G (2008a) The effect of heat waves on mental health in a temperate Australian city. *Environmental Health Perspectives* 116 (10):1369-1375.

Hansen AL, Bi P, Ryan P, Nitschke M, Pisaniello D, Tucker G (2008b) The effect of heat waves on hospital admissions for renal disease in a temperate city of Australia. *International Journal of Epidemiology* 37 (6):1359-1365.

Health Information System Development Office (2010) Soving the mystery of death: Overhaul the system of death. *Moh-Anamai* 4 (19):37-41.

Hémon D, Jougla E (2003) Surmortalité liée à la canicule d'août 2003-Rapport d'étape. Estimation de la surmortalité et principales caractéristiques épidémiologiques [Excess mortality related to the heatwave of August 2003, Progress Report, Estimation of mortality and major epidemiological characteristics]. Institut National de la Santé et de la Recherche Médicale (INSERM) Paris, France

Hollowell DR (2010) Perceptions of, and reactions to, environmental heat: A brief note on issues of concern in relation to occupational health. *Glob Health Action* 3.

Hoshiko S, English P, Smith D, Trent R (2010) A simple method for estimating excess mortality due to heat waves, as applied to the 2006 California heat wave. *International Journal of Public Health* 55 (2):133-137.

Huang W, Kan H, Kovats S (2010) The impact of the 2003 heat wave on mortality in Shanghai, China. *Science of the Total Environment* 408 (11):2418-2420.

Hunter GD (1887) Notes on heat and "heat-stroke" at Assouan in the summer of 1886. *British Medical Journal* 2 (1384):65.

Ingole V, Juvekar S, Muralidharan V, Sambhudas S, Rocklöv J (2012) The short-term association of temperature and rainfall with mortality in Vadu Health and Demographic Surveillance System: A population level time series analysis. *Global Health Action* 5 (19118):44-52.

IPCC (2001) Climate change 2001: The scientific basic. Contribution of working group I to the Third Assessment Report of the Intergovernmental Panel on Climate Change. Cambridge University Press, Cambridge, UK.

IPCC (2007) Climate change 2007: Impacts, adaptation and vulnerability. Contribution of Working Group II to the Fourth Assessment Report of the Intergovernmental Panel on Climate Change. Cambridge University Press, Cambridge, UK.

ISO (1989) Hot environments - Estimation of heat stress on working man, based on WBGT-index (wet bulb globe temperature). ISO Standard 7423. International Standards Organization, Geneva

Jaakkola JJK (2003) Case-crossover design in air pollution epidemiology. *European Respiratory Journal, Supplement* 21 (40):81S-85S.

Jackson JE, Yost MG, Karr C, Fitzpatrick C, Lamb BK, Chung SH, Chen J, Avise J, Rosenblatt RA, Fenske RA (2010) Public health impacts of climate change in Washington State: Projected mortality risks due to heat events and air pollution. *Climatic Change* 102:159-186.

Jakreng C (2010) Physical health effects from occupational exposure to natural heat among salt production workers in Samutsonghram province. Srinakharinwirot university, Bangkok

Janes H, Sheppard L, Lumley T (2005a) Case-crossover analyses of air pollution exposure data: Referent selection strategies and their implications for bias. *Epidemiology* 16 (6):717-726.

Janes H, Sheppard L, Lumley T (2005b) Overlap bias in the case-crossover design, with application to air pollution exposures. *Statistics in Medicine* 24 (2):285-300.

Kaiser R, Le Tertre A, Schwartz J, Gotway CA, Daley WR, Rubin CH (2007) The effect of the 1995 heat wave in Chicago on all-cause and cause-specific mortality. *American Journal of Public Health* 97 Suppl 1:S158-162.

Kaiser R, Rubin CH, Henderson AK, Wolfe MI, Kieszak S, Parrott CL, Adcock M (2001) Heat-related death and mental illness during the 1999 Cincinnati heat wave. *American Journal of Forensic Medicine and Pathology* 22 (3):303-307.

Kalkstein LS (1993) Health and climate change - Direct impacts in cities. *The Lancet* 342 (8884):1397-1399.

Kalkstein LS, Greene JS (1997) An evaluation of climate/mortality relationships in large U.S. cities and the possible impacts of a climate change. *Environmental Health Perspectives* 105 (1):84-93.

Katsouyanni K, Pantazopoulou A, Touloumi G, Tselepidaki I, Moustris K, Asimakopoulos D, Poulopoulou G, Trichopoulos D (1993) Evidence for interaction between air pollution and high temperature in the causation of excess mortality. *Archives Envionmental Health* 48 (4):235-242.

Keatinge WR, Coleshaw SRK, Easton JC, Cotter F, Mattock MB, Chelliah R (1986) Increased in platelet and red cells counts, blood viscosity, and plasma cholesterol level during heat stress, and mortality from coronary and cerebral thrombosis. *American Journal of Medicine* 81 (5):795-800.

Keatinge WR, Donaldson GC, Cordioli E, Martinelli M, Kunst AE, Mackenbach JP, Nayha S, Vuori I (2000) Heat related mortality in warm and cold regions of Europe: Observational study. *BMJ* 321 (7262):670-673.

Kelly M, Strazdins L, Dellora T, Seubsman S, Sleigh A (2010) Thailand's work and health transition. *International Labour Review* 149 (3):373-386.

Kenney WL, Munce TA (2003) Invited review: Aging and human temperature regulation. *Journal of Applied Physiology* 95 (6):2598-2603.

Kilbourne EM (2002) Heat-related illness: Current status of prevention efforts. *American Journal of Preventive Medicine* 22 (4):328-329.

Kilbourne EM, Choi K, Jones TS, Thacker SB (1982) Risk factors for heatstroke. A case-control study. *Journal of the American Medical Association* 247 (24):3332-3336.

Kim H, Ha JS, Park J (2006) High temperature, heat index, and mortality in 6 major cities in South Korea. *Archives of Environmental and Occupational Health* 61 (6):265-270.

Kinney PL, O'Neill MS, Bell ML, Schwartz J (2008) Approaches for estimating effects of climate change on heat-related deaths: Challenges and opportunities. *Environmental Science & Policy* 11 (1):87-96.

Kjellstrom T Climate change, heat exposure and labour productivity. In: The 12th Conference of the International Society for Environmental Epidemiology (ISEE), Buffalo, USA, 19-23 August 2000. vol 4. Epidemiology, p S144

Kjellstrom T (2009a) Climate change exposures, chronic disease and mental health in urban populations: A threat to health security, particularly for the poor and disadvantaged. World Health Organization, Kobe, Japan. http://www.who.int/kobe_centre/publications/cc_work_ability.pdf. Accessed 7 March 2012

Kjellstrom T (2009b) Editorial: Climate change, direct heat exposure, health and well-being in low and middle-income countries. *Global Health Action* 2.

Kjellstrom T, Butler AJ, Lucas RM, Bonita R (2010) Public health impact of global heating due to climate change: Potential effects on chronic non-communicable diseases. *International Journal of Public Health* 55:97-103.

Kjellstrom T, Crowe J (2011) Climate change, workplace heat exposure, and occupational health and productivity in Central America. *International Journal of Occupational and Environmental Health* 17 (3):270-281.

Kjellstrom T, Gabrysch S, Lemke B, Dear K (2009a) The "Hothaps" program for assessing climate change impacts on occupational health and productivity: An invitation to carry out field studies *Global Health Action* 2.

Kjellstrom T, Holmer I, Lemke B (2009b) Workplace heat stress, health and productivity - an increasing challenge for low and middle-income countries during climate change. *Global Health Action* 2.

Kjellstrom T, Kovats RS, Lloyd SJ, Holt T, Tol RS (2009c) The direct impact of climate change on regional labor productivity. *Archives of Environmental and Occupational Health* 64 (4):217-227.

Kjellstrom T, Weaver H (2009) Climate change and health: Impacts, vulnerability, adaptation and mitigation. *NSW Public Health Bulletin* 20 (2):5-9.

Knowlton K, Rotkin-Ellman M, King G, Margolis HG, Smith D, Solomon G, Trent R, English P (2009) The 2006 California heat wave: Impacts on hospitalizations and emergency department visits. *Environmental Health Perspective* 117 (1):61-67.

Koppe C, Kovats RS, Jendritzky G, Menne B (2004) Heat-waves: Risks and responses. World Health Organization. World Health Organization Regional Office for Europe, Geneva, Switzerland. 2

Kovats RS, Akhtar R (2008) Climate, climate change and human health in Asian cities. *Environment and Urbanization* 20 (1):165-175.

Kovats RS, Hajat S (2008) Heat stress and public health: A critical review. *Annual Review of Public Health* 29 (9):41-55.

Kovats RS, Kristie LE (2006) Heatwaves and public health in Europe. *European Journal of Public Health* 16 (6):592-599.

Kunst AE, Looman CWN, Mackenbach JP (1993) Outdoor air temperature and mortality in The Netherlands: A time-series analysis. *American Journal of Epidemiology* 137 (3):331-341.

Kwok JSS, Chan TYK (2005) Recurrent heat-related illnesses during antipsychotic treatment. *Annals of Pharmacotherapy* 39 (11):1940-1942.

Langkulsen U (2011) Climate change and occupational health in Thailand. *Asian-Pacific Newsletter on Occupational Health and Safety* 18 (1):12-13.

Langkulsen U, Vichit-Vadakan N, Taptagaporn S (2010) Health impact of climate change on occupational health and productivity in Thailand. *Global Health Action* 3.

Lemke B, Kjellstrom T (2012) Calculating workplace WBGT from meteorological data: A tool for climate change assessment. *Industrial Health* 50 (4):267-278.

Lepeule J, Rondeau V, Filleul L, Dartigues JF (2006) Survival analysis to estimate association between short-term mortality and air pollution. *Environmental Health Perspectives* 114 (2):242-247.

Levy D, Lumley T, Sheppard L, Kaufman J, Checkoway H (2001) Referent selection in case-crossover analyses of acute health effects of air pollution. *Epidemiology* 12 (2):186-192.

Liljegren JC, Carhart RA, Lawday P, Tschopp S, Sharp R (2008) Modeling the wet bulb globe temperature using standard meteorological measurements. *Journal of Occupational and Environmental Hygiene* 5 (10):645-655.

Limsakul A, Goes JI (2008) Empirical evidence for interannual and longer period variability in Thailand surface air temperatures. *Atmospheric Research* 87 (2):89-102.

Liu L, Breitner S, Pan X, Franck U, Leitte AM, Wiedensohler A, von Klot S, Wichmann HE, Peters A, Schneider A (2011a) Associations between air temperature and cardio-respiratory mortality in the urban area of Beijing, China: A time-series analysis. *Environmental Health* 10:51.

Liu L, Zhou Y, Zhang J (2011b) A case-crossover study: The effects of heat waves on daily mortality caused by respiratory disease in Beijing. *Epidemiology* 22 (1):S23-S24

Loughnan ME, Nicholls N, Tapper NJ (2010) The effects of summer temperature, age and socioeconomic circumstance on acute myocardial infarction admissions in Melbourne, Australia. *International Journal of Health Geographics* 9 (1):41.

Lu Y, Symons JM, Geyh AS, Zeger SL (2008) An approach to checking case-crossover analyses based on equivalence with time-series methods. *Epidemiology* 19 (2):169-175.

Lu Y, Zeger SL (2007) On the equivalence of case-crossover and time series methods in environmental epidemiology. *Biostatistics* 8 (2):337-344.

Lumlertgul D, Chuaychoo B, Thitiarchakul S, Srimahachota S, Sangchun K, Keoplung M (1992) Heat stroke-induced multiple organ failure. *Renal Failure* 14 (1):77-80.

Maclure M (1991) The case-crossover design: A method for studying transient effects on the risk of acute events. *American Journal of Epidemiology* 133 (2):144-153.

Macpherson RK (1960) Physiological responses to hot environments - an account of work done in Singapore, 1948-1953. Royal Naval Tropical Research Unit. Medical Research Council, Special Report Series No. 298.

Marks D (2011) Climate change and Thailand: Impact and response. *Contemporary Southeast Asia* 33 (2):229-258.

Martens W (1998) Climate change, thermal stress and mortality changes. *Social Science and Medicine* 46 (3):331-344.

Martin SL, Cakmak S, Hebbern CA, Avramescu ML, Tremblay N (2012) Climate change and future temperature-related mortality in 15 Canadian cities. *International Journal of Biometeorology* 56 (4):605-619.

Mathee A, Oba J, Rose A (2010) Climate change impacts on working people (the HOTHAPS initiative): Findings of the South African pilot study. *Global Health Action* 3.

McGeehin MA, Mirabelli M (2001) The potential impacts of climate variability and change on temperature-related morbidity and mortality in the United States. *Environmental Health Perspectives* 109 (2 Suppl):185-189.

McMichael AJ, Campbell-Lendrum D, Corvalan CF, Ebi KL, Githeko A, Scheraga JD, Woodward A (2003) Climate change and human health: Risks and responses. World Health Organization, Geneva.

McMichael AJ, Githeko A (2001) Human health. In: Climate change 2001: Impacts, adaptation, and vulnerability. Contribution of Working Group II to the Third Assessment Report of the Intergovernmental Panel on Climate Change Cambridge University Press, Cambridge, UK.

McMichael AJ, Patz JA, Kovats RS (1998) Impacts of global environmental change on future health and health care in tropical countries. *British Medical Bulletin* 54 (2):475-488.

McMichael AJ, Wilkinson P, Kovats RS, Pattenden S, Hajat S, Armstrong B, Vajanapoom N, Niciu EM, Mahomed H, Kingkeow C, Kosnik M, O'Neill MS, Romieu I, Ramirez-Aguilar M, Barreto ML, Gouveia N, Nikiforov B (2008) International study of temperature, heat and urban mortality: The 'ISOTHURM' project. *International Journal of Epidemiology* 37 (5):1121-1131.

McMichael AJ, Woodruff RE, Hales S (2006) Climate change and human health: present and future risks. *The Lancet* 367 (9513):859-869.

McNeil M The Torrid Zone: Now and in the future. In: Life in the Torrid World Symposium, Cairns, Australia, August 2009.

Medina-Ramon M, Zanobetti A, Cavanagh DP, Schwartz J (2006) Extreme temperatures and mortality: Assessing effect modification by personal characteristics and specific cause of death in a multi-city case-only analysis. *Environmental Health Perspectives* 114 (9):1331 - 1336.

Meteorological Development Bureau (2010) Daily weather data. Thai Meteorological Department, Ministry of Information and Communication Technology, Bangkok, Thailand

Meteorological Development Bureau (2012) The climate of Thailand. Climatological Group, Meteorological Development Bureau, Thai Meteorological Department, Bangkok, Thailand, 1-7. http://www.tmd.go.th/en/archive/thailand_climate.pdf. January 2012

Metzger KB, Ito K, Matte TD (2009) Summer heat and mortality in New York city: How hot is too hot? *Environmental Health Perspectives* 118 (1).

Mittleman MA, Maclure M, Robins JM (1995) Control sampling strategies for case-crossover studies: An assessment of relative efficiency. *American Journal of Epidemiology* 142 (1):91-98.

MMWR (1984) Centers for Disease Control and Prevention (CDC). Fatalities from occupational heat exposure. *Morbidity and Mortality Weekly Report* July 20, 33 (28):410-412.

MMWR (1995) Centers for Disease Control and Prevention (CDC). Heat-related mortality -- Chicago, July 1995. *Morbidity and Mortality Weekly Report* August 44 (31):577-579.

MMWR (2008) Centers for Disease Control and Prevention (CDC). Heat-related deaths among crop workers - United States, 1992-2006. *Morbidity and Mortality Weekly Report* June 20, 57 (24):649-653.

Morabito M, Cecchi L, Crisci A, Modesti PA, Orlandini S (2006) Relationship between work-related accidents and hot weather conditions in Tuscany (Central Italy). *Industrial Health* 44:458-464.

Nag PK, Nag A, Ashtekar SP (2007) Thermal limits of men in moderate to heavy work in tropical farming. *Industrial Health* 45:107-117.

National Economic and Social Development Board (2007) Population Projections for Thailand 2000 - 2030. National Economic and Social Development Board, Bangkok, Thailand.

National Statistical Office (2011) The preliminary report of 2010 population and housing census. Ministry of Information and Communication Technology, Bangkok, Thailand. http://popcensus.nso.go.th/upload/census-report-6-4-54.pdf.

National Statistical Office (2012) Report of the labour force survey. September 2012. Ministry of Information and Communication Technology, Bangkok, Thailand. http://service.nso.go.th/nso/nsopublish/themes/files/lfs55/reportSep.pdf.

National Weather Service (2012) Maximum heat index forecasts. National Oceanic and Atmospheric Administration (NOAA), Maryland http://www.hpc.ncep.noaa.gov/heat_index_MAX.shtml. Accessed 14 December 2012

Navidi W (1998) Bidirectional case-crossover designs for exposures with time trends. *Biometrics* 54 (2):596-605.

Navidi W, Weinhandl E (2002) Risk set sampling for case-crossover designs. *Epidemiology* 13 (1):100-105.

Nitschke M, Tucker GR, Hansen AL, Williams S, Zhang Y, Bi P (2011) Impact of two recent extreme heat episodes on morbidity and mortality in Adelaide, South Australia: A case-series analysis. *Environmental Health: A Global Access Science Source* 10:42.

O'Neill MS, Zanobetti A, Schwartz J (2005) Disparities by race in heat-related mortality in four US cities: The role of air conditioning prevalence. *Journal of Urban Health* 82 (2):191-197.

Oechsli FW, Buechley RW (1970) Excess mortality associated with three Los Angeles September hot spells. *Environmental Research* 3 (4):277-284.

Office of Natural Resources and Environmental Policy and Planning (2009) National strategy on climate change management B.E. 2551-2555 (A.D. 2008-2012). Ministry of Natural Resources and Environemnt, Thailand, Bangkok.

Oke TR (1973) City size and the urban heat island. *Atmospheric Environment* 7 (8):769-779.

OSHA (2005) OSHA best practices for hospital-based first receivers of victims from mass casualty incidents involving the release of hazardous substances Occupational Safety and Health Administration, Washington, DC

Ostro B, Rauch S, Green R, Malig B, Basu R (2010) The effects of temperature and use of air conditioning on hospitalizations. *American Journal of Epidemiology* 172 (9):1053-1061.

Page LA, Hajat S, Kovats RS (2007) Relationship between daily suicide counts and temperature in England and Wales. *Britis Journal of Psychiatry* 191:106-112.

Pandolf KB (1997) Aging and human heat tolerance. *Experimental Aging Research* 23 (1):69-105.

Parsons K (2003) Human thermal environments: The effects of hot, moderate, and cold environments on human health, comfort and performance. 2nd edn. Taylor & Francis, London.

Parsons K (2009) Maintaining health, comfort and productivity in heat waves. *Glob Health Action* 2.

Patz JA, Campbell-Lendrum D, Gibbs H, Woodruff R (2008) Health impact assessment of global climate change: Expanding on comparative risk assessment approaches for policy making. *Annual Review of Public Health* 29:27-39.

Patz JA, Campbell-Lendrum D, Holloway T, Foley JA (2005) Impact of regional climate change on human health. *Nature* 438 (7066):310-317.

Patz JA, Engelberg D, Last J (2000) The effects of changing weather on public health. *Annual Review of Public Health* 21:271-307.

Piver WT, Ando M, Ye F, Portier CJ (1999) Temperature and air pollution as risk factors for heat stroke in Tokyo, July and August 1980-1995. *Environmental Health Perspectives* 107 (11):911.

Pudpong N, Hajat S (2011) High temperature effects on out-patient visits and hospital admissions in Chiang Mai, Thailand. *Science of the Total Environment* 409:5260–5267.

Ramsay T, Burnett R, Krewski D (2003) Exploring bias in a generalized additive model for spatial air pollution data. *Environmental Health Perspectives* 111 (10):1283-1288.

Ramsey JD (1995) Task performance in heat: A review. *Ergonomics* 38:154-165.

Ramsey JD, Burford CL, Beshir MY, Jensen RC (1983) Effects of workplace thermal conditions on safe work behavior. *Journal of Safety Research* 14 (3):105-114.

Ren C, Williams GM, Mengersen K, Morawska L, Tong S (2009) Temperature enhanced effects of ozone on cardiovascular mortality in 95 large US communities, 1987-2000: Assessment using the NMMAPS data. *Archives of Environmental and Occupational Health* 64 (3):177-184.

Ren C, Williams GM, Morawska L, Mengersen K, Tong S (2008) Ozone modifies associations between temperature and cardiovascular mortality: Analysis of the NMMAPS data. *Occupational and Environmental Medicine* 65 (4):255-260.

Riedel D (2004) Chapter 9: Human health and well-being. Climate change impacts and adaptation: A Canadian perspective. Natural Resources Canada, Ottawa.

Robine J-M, Cheung SLK, Roy SL, Oyen HV, Griffiths C, Michel J-P, Herrmann FR (2008) Death toll exceeded 70,000 in Europe during the summer of 2003. *Comptes Rendus Biologies* 331 (2):171-178.

Rocklov J, Forsberg B (2008) The effect of temperature on mortality in Stockholm 1998-2003: A study of lag structures and heatwave effects. *Scandinavian Journal of Public Health* 36 (5):516-523.

Rocklov J, Forsberg B (2010) The effect of high ambient temperature on the elderly population in three regions of Sweden. *International Journal of Environmental Research and Public Health* 7 (6):2607-2619.

Seubsman S-A, Yiengprugsawan V, Sleigh A, the Thai Cohort Study Team (2012) A large national Thai Cohort Study of health-risk transition based on Sukhothai Thammathirat Open University students. *ASEAN Journal Open Distance Learn.* 41(1):1-11.

Schifano P, Cappai G, De Sario M, Michelozzi P, Marino C, Bargagli A, Perucci C (2009) Susceptibility to heat wave-related mortality: A follow-up study of a cohort of elderly in Rome. *Environmental Health* 8 (1):50.

Schrier RW, Hano J, Keller HI, Finkel RM, Gilliland PF, Cirksena WJ, Teschan PE (1970) Renal, metabolic, and circulatory responses to heat and exercise. *Annals of Internal Medicine* 73 (2):213-223.

Schwartz J (2005) Who is sensitive to extremes of temperature?: A case-only analysis. *Epidemiology* 16 (1):67-72.

Schwartz J, Dockery DW (1992) Increased mortality in Philadelphia associated with daily air pollution concentrations. *American Review of Respiratory Disease* 145 (3):600-604.

SEA START RC (2009) Future Climate Projection for Thailand and Mainland Southeast Asia Using PRECIS and ECHAM4 Climate Models. In: Chinvanno S, Laung-Aram V, Sangmanee C et al. (eds) Southeast Asia START Regional Centre Technical Report No. 18

Semenza JC, McCullough JE, Flanders WD, McGeehin MA, Lumpkin JR (1999) Excess hospital admissions during the July 1995 heat wave in Chicago. *American Journal of Preventive Medicine* 16 (4):269-277.

Semenza JC, Rubin CH, Falter KH, Selanikio JD, Flanders WD, Howe HL, Wilhelm JL (1996) Heat-related deaths during the July 1995 heat wave in Chicago. *New England Journal of Medicine* 335 (2):84-90.

Sheffield PE, Landrigan PJ (2011) Global climate change and children's health: Threats and strategies for prevention. *Environmental Health Perspectives* 119 (3):291-298.

Sintunawa C, Zhang J, Rajbhandari PCL, Jungrungrueng S (2009) Bangkok assessment report on climate change 2009. Bangkok Metropolitan Administration, Green Leaf Foundation and United Nations Environment Programme, Bangkok, 90.

Sirisawang S (2011) Heat wave and undefined deaths. Thai Environmental Corporation Foundation, Bangkok, Thailand. http://www.envcorpthai.com/news/detail.php?id=38%20acess. Accessed 1 August 2011

Sleigh A, Seubsman S, Bain C, Thai Cohort Team (2008) Cohort profile: the Thai cohort of 87,134 open university students. *International Journal of Epidemiology* 37:266-272.

Sohar E (1982) Men, microclimate and society: Physiological requirements of the human body for comfortable indoor climate. *Energy and Buildings* 4 (2):149-154.

Steadman RG (1979) The assessment of sultriness. Part I: A temperature-humidity index based on human physiology and clothing science. *Journal of Applied Meteorology* 18 (7):861-873.

Steadman RG (1984) A universal scale of apparent temperature. *Journal of Climate & Applied Meteorology* 23 (12):1674-1687.

Sutthanusorn P, Miller CR, Sa-nguankulchai S, Bober S, Charoensiri G, Harrison D, Hickcox R (2012) Heat impacts on occupational health. Thammasat University, Bangkok. http://heatisthesilentkiller.weebly.com/.

Tawatsupa B, Dear K, Kjellstrom T, Sleigh A (2012a) The association between temperature and mortality in tropical middle income Thailand from 1999 to 2008. *International Journal of Biometeorology* (ICB 2011-Students/new professionals):1-13.

Tawatsupa B, Lim LL-Y, Kjellstrom T, Seubsman S, Sleigh A, the Thai Cohort Study team (2010) The association between overall health, psychological distress, and occupational heat stress among a large national cohort of 40,913 Thai workers. *Global Health Action* 3.

Tawatsupa B, Lim LL-Y, Kjellstrom T, Seubsman S, Sleigh A, the Thai Cohort Study team (2012b) Association between occupational heat stress and kidney disease among 37,816 workers in the Thai Cohort Study (TCS). *Journal of Epidemiology* 22 (3):251-260.

Tawatsupa B, Yiengprugsawan V, Kjellstrom T, Berecki-Gisolf J, Seubsman S-A, Sleigh A (2013) The association between heat stress and occupational injury among Thai workers: finding of the Thai Cohort Study. *Industrial Health* 51 (1):34-46.

Tawatsupa B, Yiengprugsawan V, Kjellstrom T, Seubsman S-a, Sleigh A, the Thai Cohort Study Team (2012c) Heat stress, health, and wellbeing: findings from a large national cohort of Thai adults. *BMJ Open* 2 (6):e001396.

Thai Meteorological Department (2007) Climate change in Thailand for last 52 years. Thai Meteorological Department, Bangkok, Thailand. http://www.tmd.go.th/info/info.php?FileID=86. Accessed 4 February 2012

Thai Meteorological Department (2009) Future climate change projection in Thailand. Thai Meteorological Department, Bangkok, Thailand. http://www.tmd.go.th/programs/uploads/intranet/DOCS/ncct-0008.pdf. Accessed September 2009

Tong S, Ren C, Becker N (2010) Excess deaths during the 2004 heatwave in Brisbane, Australia. *International Journal of Biometeorology* 54 (4):393-400.

Vajanapoom N, Shy CM, Neas LM, Loomis D (2002) Associations of particulate matter and daily mortality in Bangkok, Thailand. *Southeast Asian Journal of Tropical Medicine and Public Health* 33 (2):389-399.

Vaneckova P, Beggs PJ, de Dear RJ, McCracken KWJ (2008) Effect of temperature on mortality during the six warmer months in Sydney, Australia, between 1993 and 2004. *Environmental Research* 108 (3):361-369.

Vichit-Vadakan N, Vajanapoom N, Ostro B (2008) The public health and air pollution in Asia (PAPA) project: Estimating the mortality effects of particulate matter in Bangkok, Thailand. *Environmental Health Perspectives* 116 (9):1179-1182.

Vichit-Vadakan N, Vajanapoom N, Ostro B (2010) Part 3. Estimating the effects of air pollution on mortality in Bangkok, Thailand. *Research Report/Health Effects Institute* (154):231-268.

Victorian Government Department of Human Services (2009) January 2009 heatwave in Victoria: An assessment of health impacts. the Victorian Government Department of Human Services, Melbourne, Victoria.

Wang SV, Coull BA, Schwartz J, Mittleman MA, Wellenius GA (2011a) Potential for bias in case-crossover studies with shared exposures analyzed using SAS. *American Journal of Epidemiology* 174 (1):118-124.

Wang XY, Barnett AG, Yu W, FitzGerald G, Tippett V, Aitken P, Neville G, McRae D, Verrall K, Tong S (2011b) The impact of heatwaves on mortality and emergency hospital admissions from non-external causes in Brisbane, Australia. *Occupational and Environmental Medicine* 69 (3):163-169.

Weiner JS, Khogali M (1980) A physiological body-cooling unit for treatment of heat stroke. *The Lancet* 315 (8167):507–509.

Wichmann J, Andersen Z, Ketzel M, Ellermann T, Loft S (2011) Apparent temperature and cause-specific emergency hospital admissions in greater Copenhagen, Denmark. *PLoS ONE* 6 (7):e22904.

Wilby RL (2003) Past and projected trends in London's urban heat island. *Weather* 58 (7):251-260.

Williams S, Nitschke M, Weinstein P, Pisaniello DL, Parton KA, Bi P (2012) The impact of summer temperatures and heatwaves on mortality and morbidity in Perth, Australia 1994-2008. *Environment International* 40 (1):33-38.

Wong CM, Vichit-Vadakan N, Vajanapoom N, Ostro B, Thach TQ, Chau PY, Chan EK, Chung RY, Ou CQ, Yang L, Peiris JS, Thomas GN, Lam TH, Wong TW, Hedley AJ, Kan H, Chen B, Zhao N, London SJ, Song G, Chen G, Zhang Y, Jiang L, Qian Z, He Q, Lin HM, Kong L, Zhou D, Liang S, Zhu Z, Liao D, Liu W, Bentley CM, Dan J, Wang B, Yang N, Xu S, Gong J, Wei H, Sun H, Qin Z (2010) Part 5. Public health and air pollution in Asia (PAPA): A combined analysis of four studies of air pollution and mortality. *Research Report/Health Effects Institute* (154):377-418.

World Health Organization (1946) Preamble to the constitution of the World Health Organization as adopted by the International Health Conference, New York, 19-22 June, 1946; signed on 22 July 1946 by the representatives of 61 States (Official Records of the World Health Organization, no. 2, p. 100) and entered into force on 7 April 1948.

World Health Organization (1993) International statistical classification of diseases and related health problems. Tenth Revision. World Health Organization, Geneva, Switzerland.

World Health Organization (2010) Protecting human health from climate change: Report of the technical discussions, 18-21 August 2009. World Health Organization, Regional Office for South-East Asia, New Delhi.

Wyndham CH (1965) A survey of the causal factors in heat stroke and of their prevention in the gold mining industry. *Journal of the South African Institute of Mining and Metallurgy* 66:125-155.

Wyndham CH (1969) Adaptation to heat and cold. *Environmental Research Letters* 2 (5-6):442-469.

Wyndham CH, Benade AJA, Williams CG, Strydom NB, Goldin A, Heyns AJA (1968) Changes in central circulation and body fluid spaces during acclimatization to heat. *Journal of Applied Physiology* 25 (5):586-593.

Yaglou CP, Minard D (1957) Control of heat casualties at military training centers. *American Medical Association Archives of Industrial Health* 16 (4):302-316.

Ye X, Wolff R, Yu W, Vaneckova P, Pan X, Tong S (2012) Ambient temperature and morbidity: A review of epidemiological evidence. *Environmental Health Perspectives* 120 (1):19-28.

Ingram Content Group UK Ltd.
Milton Keynes UK
UKHW010851060623
422954UK00001B/180